reclaiming a lost soul

Codependency
Revealed & Recovered

A Guide for Mental Health
Practitioners and Their Clients

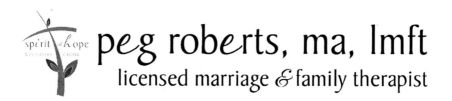

spirit of hope
COUNSELING CENTER

peg roberts, ma, lmft
licensed marriage & family therapist

Wasteland Press

www.wastelandpress.net
Shelbyville, KY USA

Reclaiming a Lost Soul:
Codependency Revealed & Recovered:
A Guide for Mental Health Practitioners and Their Clients
by Peg Roberts, MA, LMFT
President & Clinical Director
Spirit of Hope Counseling Center

First printing – November 2013
ISBN: 978-1-60047-913-7
Library of Congress Control Number: 2013951380

Cover Design by: Sarah Shattuck, Four Seasons Design Company
Editor: Andrea Bandle
Interior Design: Peg Roberts

Printed in the U.S.A.

0   1   2   3   4   5   6   7   8   9   10   11   12   13   14

For book sales, please contact
Spirit of Hope Counseling Center
Spiritofhopecc.com
952-546-5565
13911 Ridgedale Drive, Suite 490
Minnetonka, MN 55305

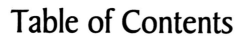

Table of Contents

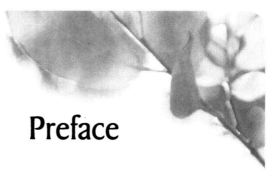

Preface

Thank you for your interest in helping to reclaim lost souls. As mental health practitioners, our goal is to be able to help people find their true selves and learn to be the person they were meant to be...to be authentic. We know that many people have had difficult lives and their souls and sense of self have gotten lost along the way.

Codependency has hurt many people and we, as therapists, need to know how to help them. For some people, codependency has destroyed their lives and for others even caused their death (from suicide and severe depression). We can't minimize the effects on individuals and families. Due to the subtleness of the issue, we must be aware of the symptoms and provide expert help for our clients.

Codependency healing, like many other psychological issues, is not a destination but an ongoing journey. Its recovery takes time and can be something clients will learn to manage their entire lives. What I've seen, however, is the relief and hope my clients gain as we work through their issues, learn new strategies for healthier relationships, and help them take back the power they have given away and the soul they have lost.

When I talk about losing souls, what that means is that people have given up themselves: their thoughts, dreams, emotions, and even their bodies, to other people. The sense of knowing who they are gets lost. I believe it's not gone forever, however. We just need to help them find themselves again, learn to nurture themselves and eventually help them reclaim their souls. When they go through this process and become authentically who they were meant to be, they will find peace, understanding and acceptance.

I believe our soul is the essence of who we are; which, in my mind, includes our thoughts, our personality, our emotions, and the spiritual gifts we are given by God. Because of dysfunction, pain, betrayal, and trauma, however, we have given up ourselves for the sake of saving others. We survive, but we aren't sure who we are, what we want, or what meaning our lives have because our focus has been externally focused. Some of us believe we are supposed to neglect our needs only to care for loved ones. But, as therapists, we know that when we do that, we eventually get to a place of unhappiness, resentment, anger, sadness and pain. So take this time to reassess your "self" and see if you've nurtured it and claimed it as your own. Or have you given up your life only to realize how unhappy you have become?

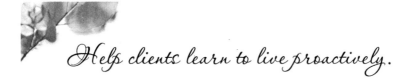

Help clients learn to live proactively.

There are strategies I've outlined throughout my book which may have been developed by other therapists and experts. For some of those examples, I don't intentionally leave out the designers but honestly don't know where I may have found those strategies. For others where I am aware of the experts and their counseling strategies, I have acknowledged those people. All the practitioners who have come before us to help us be better therapists, we say thank you! I hope that ideas from our generation of therapists bring more help for those who need it.

I've found only one book published to help practitioners treat codependency and that book was written by Cermak in 1986, *Diagnosing and Treating Co-Dependence: A Guide for Professionals who Work with Chemical Dependents, their Spouses and Children.* There have been many books written for individuals to help understand the issue of codependency, but very little to help practitioners treat codependency. This new guide, *Reclaiming a Lost Soul: Codependency Revealed and Recovered* offers new strategies for treatment and current tools for today's codependency issues.

My hope is that therapists will find this process rewarding and will ultimately be a part of the codependency healing. I love working with clients who come in and want to address their inauthenticity, their messy relationships, the issue of losing their lives to others, and the other difficult and painful symptoms that define codependency. I always have hope for a positive outcome and believe my book can outline for you specific strategies to help your clients reclaim their lives. It can be a very rewarding experience as you see your clients grow.

Through this helpful, step-by-step process, relationships that once were failing can now be healthy, functional and satisfying. Individuals can be free of obligation and learn to set healthy boundaries and ask to get their needs met. Recovery from codependency teaches clients how to live life proactively, rather than reactively and clients can take charge of their destiny and not be fearful and incessantly watchful but feel free to be themselves.

I will share a little of my personal story of recovery from codependency. My own difficult issues are what brought me to my knees and I became a believer of a power greater than myself. My higher power is Christ and I have interspersed my Christian faith here and there throughout the book. This has been my journey. Christ may not be a part of your life or a part of your clients' lives. That's OK. There is still hope and options to help individuals, couples and families through the struggle of codependency. So take what fits and leave the rest.

We can help Reclaim Lost Souls.

For me, I believe this guide has been inspired by God and only He gets full credit. I have learned that life is much more powerful and satisfying when I rely on Him for direction. I have felt His promptings (much like I did before writing this book) and gathered ideas from God. He spoke to me through others and through inspiration that only comes from Him. His presence in my life has been powerful and so, I'm enormously grateful to Him for His guidance, His grace, His love and His power to do great things in the face of pain. I believe He has taken my pain and used it to help others and I believe my pain can be used to bring light to a dark world in which others may live. I believe God can bring hope to the hopeless and life to the dead souls. Let this guide be a light to others so join me to reclaim those lost souls!

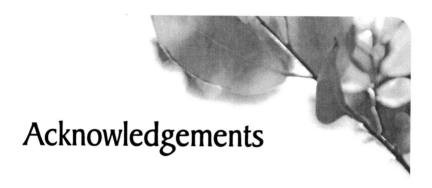

Acknowledgements

I have enormous gratitude to many people who helped me during my recovery. First, to my friend, Bev, who has been there every step of the way. She was the one I shared my week-to-week counseling with as I remembered painful memories. She listened without judgment. She was "my memory" when I was unable to remember parts of my childhood. She has been a part of my life since I was eight years old and her long-term friendship means so much to me.

I also was very fortunate to find a wonderful counselor, Linda Friel. She helped me understand my issues and took me through my difficult memories and helped me realize my abuse was more significant than I could recall. She was there when the flood of memories arrived and walked me through the pain. She helped build my self-esteem from the ground up. And to the women's therapy group Linda facilitated and I became a part of for my healing, thank you to all those women who made such an impact on my life and will always be a part of my fondest memories.

I need to thank my colleagues, Maureen Vogt, Mary Einarson, Josh Rampi (who encouraged my writing), Christina Hill, Christine Mathiowetz, Melody Richards, Kippie Palesch, Kert Stalnaker, Megan Young, Amy Kim and Dave Creek for all their support and inquisitiveness. I had several therapists ask me how I treated codependency and without their questions and encouragement, I would not have written this book. What turned into a simple outline of codependency strategies now has become what you hold in your hands. Well guys, that may have been more than you asked for, but I don't do things half way and I've agonized over this process to make it "perfect." OK, OK, maybe I need a little more codependency recovery!

Mark and Debbie Laaser are colleagues of mine and I'm honored to also call them friends. I have learned so much from them both and appreciate how they have included me in helping women who have been hurt by sexual addiction. Many of the practical skills I've offered my clients I've learned from them. Their books have been a God-send to so many people and as a therapist and codependent person, I've learned much from their writings. God has blessed them both with the power to heal broken relationships and I admire their perseverance, hard work, and dedication to the couples they help. I'm grateful they have been a part of my life as dear friends and mentors.

To my siblings, it's been great to be able to be more open and honest with one another. My oldest brother, Jim, was ten years older than I was and most of my memories don't involve him as he had moved away from home. Jim was a lost soul much of his life and had little interest in others. But I am grateful to my sister, Barb, for listening to my experiences and searching for her own truth and healthy living. She has her own personal story and has sought help to sort through her pain. And my brother, Wally, has validated my experiences and helped me remember events that seemed unreal to me. His support and understanding has brought much healing to my life. Thank you both.

My husband, Mike, needs a special thank you for standing by me for over 40 years. He was there when my journey was very painful and he was there to work on our marriage when I would have given up. His loyalty is the reason we are still married all these years. It's been a roller coaster, but we've both weathered the storm and were there together to see the light of healing. I admire him and feel so blessed to journey through life with him. His integrity and honesty mean so much to me. I want to thank him, too, for all the little things he does for me. I love him more than words can say!

You mean the world to me!

And my kids....I need to thank them so much for the love and acceptance they have given me. I know that my recovery took a toll on them when they were little and my anxiety and depression could be unpredictable. They have turned out to be wonderful adults and for that, I am eternally grateful. I only hope that the recovery their dad and I went through will be a role model for them to work on their relationships. I want them to know just how proud I am of them and how much I love them and their families.

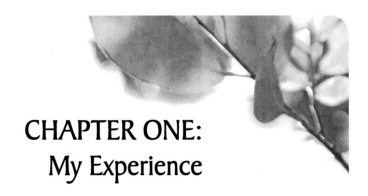

CHAPTER ONE:
My Experience

As therapists, you have heard heart-wrenching stories from your clients. So what do you do to help them? Hearing each client's story is a healing process for them. Let them talk, feel the pain, and work through those difficulties to reach that wholeness that feels so good. My story is a way of explaining how my treatment from codependency was so helpful for me. I've given you specific strategies in the following chapters that I've used over the years to help treat codependency and organized them in a way that is easy to implement. Let my story be a guide for understanding codependency and how the codependent traits and behaviors become a part of a client's life.

My story is a story of hope: hope for me, hope for you and hope for your clients. As I talk about my journey, think of yourself and how your family and life experiences have impacted you in regards to codependency and losing your soul. My background is somewhat typical of what we expect to see with codependency and alcohol abuse, but think outside the box for your clients. Think about the difficulties families' face that becomes a setup for the child to ultimately lose themselves. It may involve addictions, chronic physical or mental illness in the family and the loss of a parent where a child swoops in to take over the missing parent's role, which can be very detrimental for them. I encourage you to consider families that are emotionally, physically and spiritually absent. Here the child must learn by mistakes and hardship rather than gaining understanding from the parent who is emotionally available to teach the child what they need to know about life, morals, relationships, etc. So try to think much broader as the issues involve many other contributing factors besides addictions.

I've survived codependency. I've reclaimed my soul! I'm very grateful that I've learned healthier ways to live my life and I also realize it will be an on-going process to keep healthy. I'm grateful for the care and counsel I received through a variety of people, and my hope is that from my story you will learn to recognize this tough issue in others and provide the best intervention you can to help those people who have entrusted you with their lives. So, let's begin...

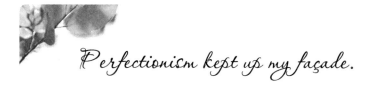

Perfectionism kept up my façade.

Like many others, codependency developed in my life at an early age. Growing up in my family was chaotic and unhealthy. Both my parents were alcoholics. I didn't know what alcoholism was at the time. I just knew I didn't like it. When I was eight years old my parents divorced. My siblings (two older brothers, ten and six years older than me, and a little sister, three years younger) and I lived with our mom full time and would visit our dad periodically, who lived three hours away. Due to the divorce, my role changed and I took on more responsibility than was healthy for me. I listened to my mom talk about the stress of finances and raising a family as a single mom. I heard my dad talk about how lonely and sad he was. It was too much for a young girl to take on and I really had no power to change anything anyway. Taking on that adult role is common in codependent households. Many children take on adult roles to "help" the family function normally (at least it feels normal!)

I thought all families had these unhealthy, dysfunctional issues. I took on a care-taking role for my mom. I would often wake up in the middle of the night and help my mother to bed after a night of drinking. I worried about her and became the parent to her while she acted like an adolescent. This was also the start of my need for control. It felt scary that people were out of control and taking charge of the situation gave me a false sense of power. What came out of that false sense of power was a self-righteous and judgmental attitude that I carried into my adult life. Many codependents try to live their lives perfectly, doing the right thing, saying the right thing. Others may view this perfectionism as haughty and preachy. This can cause major relationship issues between the one trying to do the "right" thing and their significant others.

Perfectionism takes an enormous amount of energy to keep up. I've learned that being perfect is really a facade and not a reality. There is no perfect person or perfect family. But perfectionism provided a cover-up for my guilt and shame. I believed if I looked and acted perfect and my family was perfect no one would really know how insecure and how inadequate I felt. I never thought I could measure up to others and my self-esteem was at the rock bottom. But I looked good on the outside as a mask for my inner pain. So watch for perfectionism with the clients you work with.

Much of the same issues I experienced with my mom arose in my relationship with my dad. When I visited I would spend several days with him. During that time I took care of him when he passed out at night. I cried when he cried as he said good-bye to us after a visit. And I felt falsely empowered by being "his little princess." He had opinions about how I looked and what I did and treated me like a surrogate wife. I then expected others to treat me the same way as I matured and I was very disappointed when it didn't happen. This is a real recipe for messing up a kid's thinking and their beliefs about themselves and others.

I didn't realize how much anger and resentment I carried. I felt angry at my mom for being unreasonable and unpredictable when she drank. I also didn't like her behavior and was humiliated and embarrassed by her drinking. I felt resentment towards my dad for messing up his life and in turn ultimately affecting my life. His alcoholism and "victim" mentality was a set up for me to become more responsible for him and then to become a great care-taker and I resented feeling responsible to take care of him. I felt angry much of the time. I have realized through my counseling work that many codependent people get stuck in their feelings. They might have a small range of emotion and one emotion may be their mode of operating in their life. My mode was anger. As therapists, you may find clients "stuck" in their sadness and depression, while others are stuck in the "victim" role.

With both parents alcoholic, my siblings and I learned to take care of ourselves and we all became very independent. Mom was a good cook and made great meals, except on the nights she was drinking. I honestly don't remember where my younger sister was during dinnertime as I remember making TV dinners for myself. In this environment of disconnection, I learned to keep my emotions to myself (except anger and resentment, which I freely doled out as a teen) and rarely confided in my mother or father with questions I might have had about school, relationships and sexuality. I believe this was true for my siblings, yet we never talked about this dysfunction with one another as we grew up together. We lived very separate lives. Having a supportive family to offer help and understanding was a foreign concept to me. I had learned to be a great care-taker and would provide understanding and a listening ear for both my parents. Sadly, however, no one was there for me.

As I lived through painful relationship experiences as a kid and through my teen years, I learned to be very defensive and I built a wall of protection around me so my relationships lacked emotional intimacy. Sarcasm was a way of relating to others even though it was very hurtful to everyone. I became the clown in the family and realized that I used my humor as a protective barrier to alleviate pain and insecurity and to keep people at a distance. Like most people coming into counseling, all these dynamics, all these emotions, all these experiences have had a profound, negative impact on my life.

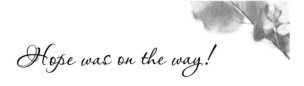

Hope was on the way!

In my mid 20's, thankfully, my mother agreed to go into treatment after our family had an intervention with her. Through her inpatient program, Al-anon was suggested for me and I was very angry and resentful to be told I needed help, since in my mind, this was my mom's problem. But after some time I realized how helpful Al-anon could be. Through the program and the wonderful people in the groups, I learned how to let go and trust God, how to focus on myself rather than the alcoholic, how to relax, and I began to understand my own codependency.

I continued with Al-anon for 15 years and found great peace and support from the program. Al-Anion's slogans and 12-Step book, *One Day at a Time*, were so helpful for me in terms of identifying my unhealthy thinking and beliefs. I lived by the slogan "One day at a time." In fact, for some time I lived "One moment at a time." These slogans and the positive reminders in the book helped me learn to live in the moment and not let my anxieties take over and focus on the future. I had no control over the future. So that understanding and change in perspective lessened my anxiety and fear. Also, the friendships and support I received helped me understand my judgmentalism and self-righteous attitude. How did that happen? Well, it was simple. Someone told me I was self-righteous! I was mad (remember I mentioned before that my default emotion was anger) and later realized I was really very hurt. It wasn't handled in the best manner, but I finally got to a place and realized that this person was right on target. So I'm grateful for the insight from another fellow Al-anon member, even though it was painful.

I also learned my parents' disease was not something I could control. It was not something I caused. And it was not something I could cure. All this brought great relief to my life. In fact, I encourage all my clients struggling with codependency to get involved in a 12-Step group of some kind. This support, I feel, moves the counseling along for the clients much quicker and more effectively.

After all those years in Al-anon I attended another codependency workshop (I attended many back then in my early 30's) when the speaker, Earnie Larsen, a codependency guru in the Minneapolis area, asked the audience the question, "If you've been in a 12-Step group for years and years, ask yourself, 'Why'?" What did he mean? I was confused. At some point I eventually realized what I think he meant was professional counseling may also be necessary for those of us "stuck" in our emotions and "stuck" in our support groups. I soon realized I needed to grow more and heal and reclaim my lost soul.

It wasn't until I hit a really depressed place in my life and felt my marriage was going to end did I finally seek out a therapist. I had read two books which had a great impact on my life. The first was Melody Beattie's book, *Codependent No More*. It was a perfect description for my struggles and when I read the book I thought she had lived my life and she felt the things I was feeling. So the information from her book brought relief for me and hope for recovery. It also normalized my experiences, thoughts and feelings. I learned that I wasn't crazy, which was a huge relief.

The other important book to me was written by John and Linda Friel, *The Secrets of Dysfunctional Families*. After attending a workshop by John Friel on their book, I realized they identified my family in a way that was helpful and it provided new information for me. This was my first introduction to therapy. Because I was feeling so depressed, angry, discouraged and afraid of everything due to anxiety, I decided to give therapy a try. My individual counseling helped address not only the dysfunction in my family of origin, but the unhealthiness in my marriage and my immediate family. It helped me identify and manage the pain and fear that arises when we live with alcoholism and abuse and how that permeates future relationships. I didn't understand how the family system impacts our present-day relationships and I began to identify that my family history was causing me pain in my present life. So I learned that I had to deal with my history as well as deal with my marriage and my emotions in the present time.

Through this process I remembered more traumas and I was devastated. As I write this, I think about how important it is for therapists to be ready for anything. Many clients have memories that have gone underground and are unavailable to the client until they are in a safe place and with a safe person with whom they can finally share their experiences. So I not only had to work on depression, anxiety, anger and fear, but now I had sexual and emotional abuse issues that I didn't recall (these memories came during a four-day intensive counseling weekend I attended) and I realized I had to face those demons as well.

Through this intensive therapy, I was able to look at my relationship with my mother and father and understand more fully how those relationships impacted my life as a child as well as my life as an adult. In therapy, I did anger work (hitting pillows in the counseling session), identified emotions and learned how to manage those emotions, as well as worked on self-esteem issues and boundary setting. I also learned I had a voice and my voice was important. Much of this self-esteem work was addressed in a weekly women's group where I had other women who understood what I had experienced, and through this intensive group work we could support one another through the painful process of healing.

From my counseling, I became aware just how much I was reacting and responding to the unhealthy values, beliefs, experiences, and decisions that had developed in my life through the lens of codependency. Once I knew what I was dealing with, I could focus on getting help and this awareness was key for me. It's a giant step to healing. Breaking through denial is a first step. Now I could learn new skills, develop new beliefs and values for myself and my family, and work towards having healthy, meaningful relationships.

Through my own recovery and from the training I've received over the years as a therapist, I realized that codependency is a very deep-seeded issue which is formed and internalized early in life and becomes the fabric of who we are. Changing it, learning new strategies to refrain from "doing life" with these ineffective ways of relating to others is a process that needs time to repair: through education, self-awareness and often professional help. You will become aware throughout this book that I encourage therapists to take their time. This life-threatening issue will take time to heal. Clients need to live life while doing therapy to address issues as they come up in the client's everyday life. It's important not to rush the process either. Clients need to be ready.

I felt very grateful that my therapist took her time with me. She always paced her therapy based on how much I could handle at the time. I did go to therapy, however, ready to work. I was very determined to rid myself of these tough emotions. I do think that all the years in Al-anon had prepared me to face the issues head on. I wanted to understand how all these experiences and beliefs made me who I was. The process, however, was very painful. It probably was the most painful time in my life. But it eventually became the pivotal point in my life where I learned about codependency, learned what feelings I was experiencing, and learned to love myself, warts and all! There is no doubt in my mind that my life was changed for the better and it then became my mission to help others who had struggled like I had.

I had much to learn about keeping a marriage intact. Many marriages in my family ended in divorce, and I acquired a faulty belief that because I was unhappy, I should leave the marriage. Thankfully, my husband believed in loyalty and he encouraged and taught me that you can work these issues out. By reaching out for help from professionals, we learned skills to communicate more effectively, learned to listen better, and we both worked on our own difficult family histories. As the pain from my childhood was processed through and I understood how those experiences impacted me, I could then let go of my anger and resentment I felt towards my husband. My marital relationship needed help, there is no doubt, but the transference of pain from my childhood relationships got in the way of a healthy connection with my husband. Some of the pain didn't belong to my husband or my marriage. It belonged in my past!

I am enormously grateful for many people who encouraged me and talked with me about faith. At an Al-Anon meeting one night, several members from the group took their precious time and talked with me about God. I learned that I was loved, no matter what I had done and no matter what was done to me. I learned I was forgiven and it was OK to forgive myself. As I grew closer to God, my heart became more and more open and I began trusting others. This took time, however, because my heart had been deeply wounded from the betrayal and pain from my past. The distancing wall I had built up around me kept me from getting close to others; but it not only kept me from the love of wonderful, supportive people, it kept me from a closer relationship with God. As I healed and started trusting trustworthy people, I learned to trust God. I was able to allow God in and believe that I could love myself as God loves me. Once the shame was lifted, I realized I did matter and what happened in my life was no longer something to be ashamed of.

This process helped me realize that sometimes we have to deal with our own pain and work through those difficult experiences before we can fully accept God's love for us. It was true for me, and may be true for many others. Initially it felt so good to believe in a Higher Power as Al-Anon teaches. But I soon realized after much searching that Christ was my Higher Power. As a child, my family didn't attend church much, but I did believe in Christ and through my healing process, I came back to my roots. My renewed faith brought so much comfort to me as I learned to pray, understand the Bible and the real love God has for me, no matter what. I believe God has compassion for all of us, no matter the situation or the choices we make. As I grew in my faith and healed from my emotional wounds, I began to forgive...forgive my parents and others who had hurt me, as well as forgive myself.

Now my experiences can help others.

My journey took me in a round-about way to a relationship with God and I know not everyone's journey will follow that same path. But God is an integral part of who I am and how I view the world. And many people come to see me for counseling because of my faith in Christ. I do realize, however, that not everyone is God centered, or even spiritual in any way. As therapists, I believe, it is our responsibility to allow each client to choose for themselves their spiritual path, and that path may be very different from yours or mine. We are to honor them in whatever their beliefs may be. I'm here to share my story and let clinicians know that sometimes we have to help clear out the clutter and pain in order for God to come into the hearts of these hurting people. If your perspective is different than mine, it's no problem. As Al-anon would tell us, "Take what you like and leave the rest." I just hope that as you help clients reclaim their souls, their worlds will open up to many people and experiences, and maybe even to God, where their lives will have more meaning and be more fulfilling.

What came out of my individual therapy, after five long years, besides relief, less anxiety, less shame and anger, was a life's direction for me professionally. I finally realized that I didn't have to be satisfied with being a wife and stay-at-home mom, even though it was the hardest and most rewarding part of my life. I could strive for more and came to believe that God had a plan for me. At the age of 40, I eventually found my way to Bethel University in St. Paul, MN after feeling called to go in to the counseling world. (I had that still, small voice within me encouraging me to go back to school. That's how God has worked in my life.) So I finished my bachelor's degree, attending school full-time as a non-traditional student, and went on at the same university to finish my Master's Degree in Counseling Psychology and completed the work to become licensed as a Marriage and Family Therapist. Wow! It took a long time. Now, after 15 years of providing therapy, I find myself training other therapists to offer hope for those in pain. I love what I'm doing and I pray that the help I bring to others, especially to those who struggle with codependency, brings hope for a bright future and healing from the wounds of addiction, neglect, mental illness and abuse.

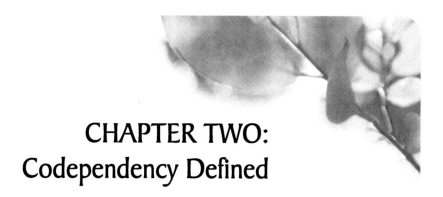

CHAPTER TWO:
Codependency Defined

As a lost soul in my 20's and 30's, I clung to those codependency experts who so well defined this issue for me. I learned that codependency develops due to learned behaviors and early experiences in the family. I don't look at the disorder as a genetic problem; however it can look that way because it develops so early, much like attachment disorders. Many children born with codependent issues are living in dysfunctional, abusive, addictive, neglectful or chronically ill (both emotionally and physically) families. We see codependency become solidified in individuals after years of unsuccessfully trying to control others' behaviors, feeling worthless, and having very unhappy, unfulfilling and exhausting relationships.

For example, due to the alcohol addiction my parents experienced, my siblings and I had little direction and guidance for our future. As a girl, I wasn't encouraged to go to college and have a career. My focus for my life was simply survival. I could only deal with the day-to-day unpredictability of my home life and it was difficult to think into the future.

Due to the lack of direction and guidance, I learned little about relationships, with men or women, and my learning took place while I was married, rather than understanding beforehand some of the dynamics couples and relationships typically go through. Rather than understand that marriage is about compromise, commitment and teamwork, I did much of the care-taking in my relationship. Because of this learned behavior, my focus in most of my relationships was on others. I was hyper-focused on my husband and my children by trying to run their lives. This controlling behavior caused lots of problems in those relationships.

I find that I still deal with some codependent behaviors and I believe it will be a life-long journey of recovery as I learn more about me, understand codependency even more than I do now, and learn to live my life rather than other people's lives.

Codependency has a consistent set of thoughts, feelings, behaviors and spiritual disconnection. The categories listed below are areas which we, as therapists, need to be acutely aware of and help define for the client so healing can be successful and satisfying. This list is in no particular order of importance. It is, however, a list that will need attention during the counseling process, moving from one issue to the next and back again.

Following is an overview of the issues to focus on. We want to look at the client's whole being, behaviors, thoughts, emotions, as well as their spirituality and sense of self. Let's look at each area in more detail. We'll begin with the behaviors that you will see and hear about in your counseling office.

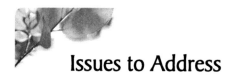

Issues to Address

BEHAVIORS

1. Compliant
2. Hyper-Vigilant
3. Neglect of Self
4. Isolated/Socially Stunted
5. Avoidant
6. Controlling
7. Reactionary
8. Perfectionism/ Overly Responsible
9. Enmeshed Relationships
10. Chameleon
11. Compulsions
12. Manipulation
13. Poor Coping Skills

THOUGHTS

1. Denial
2. Low Self-esteem
3. Black and White Thinking
4. Judgmentalism/Self - Righteousness

SPIRITUALITY/ SENSE OF SELF

1. Loss of Soul/Loss of Self
2. Spiritually Disconnected

EMOTIONS

1. Fear of Abandonment/Fear of Intimacy
2. Fear of Conflict
3. Shame/Guilt
4. Powerlessness
5. Unaware of Emotions/Emotions Out of Control

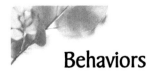

Behaviors

I. COMPLIANT

For many codependent people, they will avoid anger and rejection by giving in to the other person at the expense of their own values and integrity. Their loyalty to others becomes unhealthy as they will stay in the dysfunctional and abusive relationships for far too long. They become compliant and agreeable to others regardless of their own needs and opinions or views. They may even give in sexually to someone because of the other's perceived needs and are completely unaware of their own sexual needs. Giving up of themselves physically, by giving up their thoughts, feelings, behaviors, values, and beliefs is paramount in their mind in order to be accepted and approved by others.

Those people who are compliant are unaware of their own desires. For example, I have had many wives in my office who have found themselves in abusive relationships and done things for their husbands that they ordinarily wouldn't do. They may have been sexual in ways that were very uncomfortable for them, even painful. And yet, they have not been able to set appropriate and clear boundaries. They have been given incorrect information from their families growing up. A value that may have been demonstrated and talked about in their childhood may include the belief that good wives don't ask for things. Good wives don't say "No" to their husbands. And it's very sad that they may ultimately have given up their soul to please someone else.

2. HYPER-VIGILANT

This is a common behavior for codependents. Hyper-vigilance means being finely attuned and fearful of the environment and the people within that environment. The purpose of this behavior is to detect threats...unreal or real. The codependent can identify the problems in the room and can get overly focused, fearful, and anxious because of the awareness they have and the anxiety it provokes in them. For many, they appear nervous and jumpy, reacting to the behaviors of others in intense ways.

BEHAVIORS

1. Compliant
2. Hyper-Vigilant
3. Neglect of Self
4. Isolated/Socially Stunted
5. Avoidant
6. Controlling
7. Reactionary
8. Perfectionism/ Overly Responsible
9. Enmeshed Relationships
10. Chameleon
11. Compulsions
12. Manipulation
13. Poor Coping Skills

People with hyper-vigilance problems are difficult to be around. They scare easily, their anxiety is high, which can reverberate to others in their midst. This finely tuned-in response to fear takes an enormous amount of energy and causes exhaustion for the codependent. And their anxious behavior and fear of whatever it is, takes its toll on others around them.

3. NEGLECT OF SELF

People with codependency neglect their needs. This neglect becomes so detrimental over years that codependents can have major health problems, such as cancer, digestive problems, heart issues, etc. Ultimately it can shorten a person's life. You've probably known of someone who was a care-taker for a loved one and ultimately burned out or even died from the stress their care-taking had on them. For many, other problems develop such as unhealthy relationships, financial problems, and mental health issues (for example, depression and anxiety disorders).

Guilt and shame intermix with neglect. If they take care of themselves, they feel guilty. If they don't take care of others, they feel guilty and shameful. It's very sad and a tough issue for codependents to overcome. But it's important for them to learn to take care of their lives, their emotions, their health and their bodies.

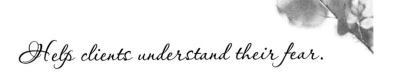

Help clients understand their fear.

4. ISOLATED/SOCIALLY STUNTED

Many codependents have difficulty managing relationships or relating to others in a healthy way. You'll often hear from codependent clients how isolated or alone they feel. For many people, adding new friends to their lives is a burden for them. They already feel overwhelmed and taking on new friends means taking on more responsibility, since they only know how to care-take.

Many people with codependency also can be very opinionated and don't mind giving others their opinions or views. They may offer unsolicited advice. Most people don't like advice or someone telling them what to do and so friendships are destroyed from these bossy and self-righteous views.

Socially, many codependents become stunted. What this means is that they have a tendency to say "No" to social events or not relate to others due to the demands or desires of the person they care-take. For example, if the codependent's loved one doesn't approve of something they desire to do, the codependent won't do it.

5. AVOIDANT

Many individuals with codependency issues use indirect and evasive communication to avoid conflict. They stay away from conflict at all costs. They also avoid or suppress their feelings and needs so as not to be too vulnerable as the vulnerability is extremely uncomfortable for them. Their ability to relate in an emotionally intimate way is a foreign concept and they may desire and ask people to get close to them, but when they do, they push those people away. Avoidance keeps all people in their lives from getting too close.

Also, many people with codependency have trouble with self-esteem and because of this, they avoid relationships. They may have anxiety and interacting with others causes so much angst and discomfort, they avoid situations to keep their anxious feelings under control. This avoidance tendency has devastating consequences in relationships and too many of these avoiders are unhappy and reclusive. They just don't know how to deal with emotions, deal with life, or deal with relationships.

6. CONTROLLING

Many people with codependency feel anxious, powerless, and have a monumental need to control others and their surroundings. Controlling other people and their environment comes from a place of fear and anxiety and often therapists can trace it back to an environment in their childhood that caused anxious feelings. If a child had grown up in a chaotic environment due to alcoholism, for example, these clients learn to try and control others and situations around them as a way to relieve their fear and anxiety. They don't learn to cooperate or negotiate which are important aspects of healthy relationships.

Those people who feel a need to be in control haven't learned to cooperate or negotiate and they will find themselves in unhealthy relationships with others. Often controlling people will find partners who take on little responsibility, are compliant, and usually shut down emotionally. This relationship may work for the couple for a while, but eventually both partners become angry and resentful towards one another.

It may seem as though a controlling person knows what they want or knows how they feel about things, however, the opposite is usually true. Many people with codependency and control issues don't really know what they personally need or desire. They tend to be so focused on others that their wants and needs are neglected. Controlling people will openly offer their advice and tell others how they "should" live or how they "should" feel. This controlling behavior is manipulative and degrading to others who are the recipients and people tend to run away from them.

"Compulsive codependents inevitably end up being controlled by the very people they attempt to control." Sandra Wilson

Many controlling individuals believe their loved ones are incapable of caring for themselves. They believe their way of doing things is the right way and others should manage their lives as they do. This gives the codependent a false sense of power (even though they really have no power over others) and can breed self-righteousness. Self-righteousness is a judgmental way of looking at others and the controlling person feels "right" in their perspective.

Controlling others seems to serve several purposes: It gives the individual a false sense of power over others and their environment; it appears to alleviate uncomfortable feelings of anxiety; and it also keeps people at a distance. All of these ways of relating are unhealthy and lack true, healthy emotional intimacy.

7. REACTIONARY

Codependents are reactionary, rather than being proactive. For many, they are great at putting out fires that arise. So living on "high alert" is familiar. Because they are so overloaded with responsibility and anxiety, they cannot keep ahead of issues. This reactionary behavior keeps the codependent person hyper-vigilant to their surroundings and ultimately does not allow them to take charge of their own life because they are overly concerned about what might happen.

These people tend to live in chaos, feel comfortable with craziness in their lives, and will even "stir the pot," so to speak, to keep their relationships in an upheaval because that chaos feels normal to them. Helping clients learn to relax, take charge of their lives and not be so overly concerned about their loved ones can be challenging. But we can help them become aware of their reactivity and teach them new ways to become proactive as well as teach them to live calmly and without drama.

8. PERFECTIONISM/OVERLY RESPONSIBLE

As a way to alleviate their anxiety, guilt and shame, many codependent people have become perfectionistic. If they can look perfect, act perfect, have the perfect life, perfect children or have a perfect home, then all is well in their world. Their anxiety is relieved and things feel "normal" or in order when all feels perfect. But we all know there is no perfection. Trying to do everything just right is impossible.

If we look at the way our culture views beauty we see people spending millions of dollars on trying to look perfect. But everyone falls short of perfection, no matter what they try to do. What's interesting is many people cognitively know there really is no perfection, however, their hearts don't always believe it. So working on those core beliefs will be a must for therapists.

Being overly responsible and trying to be perfect go hand in hand. When someone tries to take on the responsibility of another person, doing things just so, making sure everything is "right," they are set up for failure. As they take on responsibility that doesn't even belong to them, such as another's life, they will ultimately be distressed and disappointed and the other person will feel resentful towards the codependent. So overly-responsible, perfectionistic people only find themselves disappointed, disgruntled, tired and angry.

Overly-responsible behaviors cause people to work harder and do more than sometimes they are capable or is in their best interest. They feel pressure, as if there is a weight upon their shoulders. And for many people, realizing this has been how they've lived their lives for so long, are relieved to learn all the responsibility they've carried is not really theirs. But breaking free of this behavior can be difficult.

This sense of being overly responsible is something children learn when they are put in a position of taking care of siblings, for example. You'll hear stories like, "I was in charge of my siblings while mom and dad worked," or "Because my parents were gone a lot drinking or passed out on the couch, I was responsible for my little brothers and sisters." What's sad is that those clients taking on those extra burdens so early in their lives become overly responsible into their adult life. They continue to take charge of others and take charge in situations that is not their concern at all.

For those with long-term perfectionism and overly-responsible behaviors, the results can be devastating. The stress level can cause disease and even early death due to the core belief that others can't take care of things or they have to be perfect in all they do.

9. ENMESHED RELATIONSHIPS

Enmeshed relationships are relationships in which the people are not defined or independent of one another. In codependent relationships, individuals are so emotionally and psychologically close that they cannot define who they are without the other person. Often we see enmeshed relationships between children and their parents.

If a wife is living with an alcoholic or chronically ill person and her emotional and physical needs are not being met by her partner, she will often enmesh herself with one or more child to get her adult needs met. We all know how damaging that is to the children. In this situation parents don't feel the need to deal with their issues as long as some of their needs are met by others in inappropriate ways. Sexual abuse can be bred from this enmeshment, as well as other psychologically damaging issues. Because of enmeshment, children will be stunted in their emotional growth because the needs of others do not allow the child to grow emotionally. What happens is that the natural progression of independence gets cut off and you may see clients who are very emotionally immature as adults. They don't have the chance to slowly detach from parents in a healthy way. The client may still be enmeshed with a parent well into their adult years, or they enmesh with another person.

You may see a client relate to a loved one in a very unhealthy way with inappropriate attachment, for example, to an abusive person or someone who continues to harm them. Their individual definition of themselves is not well-defined, thus losing themselves and their soul to others. In these situations, the enmeshed or dependent couple feels what each other feels. They have no boundaries or clear definition of each person emotionally or psychologically...no differentiation. They can't make decisions without the other's approval or input. It's an issue that needs to be addressed during the counseling process.

10. CHAMELEON

Many codependent people have the skill to "change their colors," so to speak, depending on who is in their midst. For example, I interviewed for a job many years ago and got feedback that I was "boring." However, I know that boring is not typically how people would describe me. It was my first awareness to the chameleon characteristic that I took on in that job interview. The woman I spoke with had a flat affect, was a slow thinker, and it's exactly how I described her to people I talked with about my interview. I had changed my attitude and even my demeanor to match hers.

I view this as losing oneself to the person they are trying to connect with or to the environment they find themselves in. I believe this is a way to cope in relationships where codependents want to be liked and where they want to get approval from others. However, the real essence of who they are vanishes.

People with this chameleon quality are unsure of who they are and what they want. Their behaviors become like the people around them. It can start in school with kids acting and pretending they have qualities they don't have or doing things they normally wouldn't do. We've seen people committing crimes because someone else encouraged them to do these unlawful things, so they give up their morals and values to simply be accepted. However, after all is said and done, these codependent people feel shameful for their behavior and they don't understand how they got themselves into trouble. The truth is, they didn't know who they were, and so any "color" was OK at the time.

People in unpredictable and chaotic environments feel the need to be chameleons. Generally the codependents are not the priority in the family (because the addict or chronically ill person is the priority), and they tend to blend in. As a way to cope with the dysfunctional symptoms in their family, they may act like the other family members.

As therapists, our job is to encourage these people to define themselves more clearly. We will need to help them identify what's important to them and what they desire for their lives. As they become more clear about who they are, they can learn to be proud of themselves and no longer have to blend in and become someone they are not. It's a metamorphosis and an exciting experience to have with your clients. The changes can be amazing.

11. COMPULSIONS

Compulsive behaviors are connected with feelings of anxiety and issues of control. Because much of a codependent's life feels out of control, they will often turn to compulsive behaviors.

For example, an individual may begin compulsively cleaning...cleaning over and over even though the house may not be dirty. These compulsions are a way for the individual to feel more in control in an out-of-control environment. The person may be compulsive about their kid's clothing, making sure their child is clean, neat, and looks good, which ties in with perfectionism. It seems to be a way to make sense of their environment and as a way to alleviate fear, depression, anger and other emotions.

When anxiety gets high, these unhealthy compulsions and repetitive behaviors relieve the anxiety for a time. However, over years, the repetitions may develop into more serious compulsive behaviors like counting, checking, hand-washing, etc.

Codependents feel powerful by manipulating others.

12. MANIPULATION

When children grow up with dysfunction, with few people attentive to their needs due to alcoholism, drug abuse, and other family problems that take priority over the children, these kids learn to manipulate. This manipulation can be a means to control a situation that frightens them, or it can be a way to get the attention they are desperately seeking from an absent parent. Many manipulators can lie easily, turn the truth around on others, and talk their way out of jams. When in the presence of manipulators, many people feel confused and perplexed about what just happened in their interaction with that person.

Manipulators are often passive-aggressive, meaning they may say they are willing to do something, but turn around and complain, express exasperation and may even talk their way out of their commitments. These people can be "yes" people to alleviate further conversation and to end a discussion. They can smile, seem very positive, and yet change their attitude and complain or gossip about the person they are trying to manipulate. They are "two-faced."

For children in unhealthy environments, manipulation becomes a way to get the attention they are desperately seeking and these kids learn to use manipulation as a way to get what they want. They become very smooth, cunning, and seem helpful on the outside. Their intent is to please themselves, however, not others. What they do for others may look nice to the outside world, yet underneath, it feels crazy to those who are being manipulated.

Manipulators are very indirect in their communication and don't speak honestly. They haven't learned how to express themselves in healthy ways, and manipulation became a way of interacting in their relationships. It's a very poor way of relating and causes people around them to distrust their actions and their motivations. As they portray themselves as victims, these people hope to incite guilt in others. They want others to feel sorry for them.

13. POOR COPING STRATEGIES

Due to the unhealthy coping mechanisms in the family system, codependents have not learned skills to manage their pain. For example, children growing up in families who do not talk about feelings learn that discussing those emotions is minimized, ignored, or worse, ridiculed by others, so they learn to keep quiet and stuff them. Or in a family where anger is expressed violently, children learn to cope by trying to control their environment as a way to manage their anxiety. They are terrified and find ways to manage anxiety the best they know how. For example, if they can't control or stop the abuser, they may try to control others in the family. Or they may learn to shut down and stay quiet and away from the fray. These coping strategies may have worked well for a while as a child, but as an adult in mature relationships, they cause major marital problems.

It will be important to identify these unhealthy strategies in the counseling setting and help clients learn to manage their emotions in a productive and healthy way. Some of these coping strategies can work well, but if they are done in excess and as a tactic to avoid emotions, they become unhealthy. See the following page for an overview of common poor coping strategies.

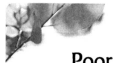

Poor Coping Strategies

- Withdrawal
- Emotional eating
- Busyness
- Workaholism
- Volunteering
- Organizing
- Controlling
- Sleeping
- Silence
- Social media
- Criticizing
- Sarcasm
- Shopping
- Gambling
- Lying
- Sexual or Emotional Affairs

- Focus on partner's recovery
- Self-righteousness
- Addictions
- Raging
- Denial
- Justifying
- Humor
- Perfectionism
- Ruminating
- TV
- Romance Novels
- Exercising
- Hyper-focused on others
- Self pity/victim role
- Anything done to excess and causing distance from others

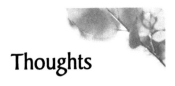

Thoughts

I. DENIAL

Denial in codependents can be as pervasive and stubborn as it is in addicts. Addicts will deny the extent of their problem, and so will codependents. Codependents will often not only deny they have a problem but deny the addict has a problem. They don't see in others how

> ### THOUGHTS
> 1. Denial
> 2. Low Self-esteem
> 3. Black and White Thinking
> 4. Judgmentalism/ Self-Righteousness

unavailable they are for them so they keep picking people in their lives who depend on them but are emotionally absent. It's very difficult to break through this denial until the codependent is ready, has a crisis, and/or feels at the end of their emotional rope. Their exhaustion can bring them in to the counseling office.

Some people in denial find it extremely difficult to ask for help. They believe they can care for themselves and have lived their lives very independently. Because they've learned that their own ways are the right ways, other people who do try to help only get resistance from the codependent. Often their pain is masked with anger, resentment, humor or isolation along with other negative coping strategies. They tend to express themselves with negativity or aggression in indirect and passive ways.

2. LOW SELF-ESTEEM

Codependent people have chronic low self-esteem and they lack assertiveness skills. They have learned that their worth is based on the views of other people. They work hard to be liked or loved, sometimes by people they don't even like. If they are not approved of by others, they believe they are unworthy and unlovable. When codependents are not clear who they are, they can change their demeanor, mood, actions, thoughts, values and beliefs easily depending on what they think others think, feel and believe.

You'll also see people with codependency having difficulty making decisions. Because they don't know what they like, dislike, or desire, they don't make decisions easily, which frustrates their family. These individuals "don't care" about where they go for dinner or they "don't care" what movie they see. They struggle with feeling as if they are doing anything "good enough" and criticize and feel shame about themselves. Many codependents value others' opinions rather than their own. Many of their needs are determined by what the other can give, even if it is very little.

3. BLACK AND WHITE THINKING

Black and white thinkers have difficulty seeing the "gray" in life. These types of people can be rigid and inflexible and their perspective on life is viewed in extremes. You will hear clients express their thoughts in ways such as, "He always does that," or "It's never going to change." This is a recipe for staying stuck in immature thought patterns and ultimately in unhealthy relationships. It's also a pattern that breeds judgmentalism and self-righteousness.

These types of people are also considered all or nothing thinkers. They view experiences as either all good or all bad. When children grow up in this rigid, right or wrong environment, they don't learn to be open and flexible. We know that people who are not flexible and fluid (changing with the ebb and flow of life) typically are unhappy and unhealthy. Life changes, whether we like it or not, and if we are not prepared for those ups and downs, we will become close-minded, inflexible and intolerant.

An important factor to consider when raising children in this environment is that shame comes from this kind of thinking. For children, they may develop a fear of making mistakes, which will cause them to believe that mistakes make them "bad." You are only good if you are perfect. Shame flourishes in this environment. Ideally, we hope to instill in our clients that mistakes or failures don't make us "bad." We just need to go back to the drawing board and figure out another option.

If families only have the good and bad mentality, favoritism can develop between parents and children. If a child is "good" and does "everything right," another child who makes mistakes can be viewed as defective and wrong. It's a very painful system to grow up in and it's also a set up for the siblings to resent that "good" child. They learn, certainly, that they will "never" measure up and may give up trying or choose unhealthy coping strategies in which to survive. Sibling competition thrives. Also, these children can become perfectionistic and overly responsible, as you'll read below, as a way to "measure up" and be seen as "good."

4. **JUDGMENTALISM/SELF-RIGHTEOUSNESS**

    Judgmentalism and self-righteousness are difficult traits to treat. For many, judging others has been a part of their family's history for a lifetime. They have complained about others as a way to feel better about themselves. When families have "black and white" thinking, they believe things are simply right or wrong and they openly share their opinion/criticism to whoever will listen. This judgmental attitude permeates the family system and the children now become judging about others as a way to communicate and connect with their parent(s).

Making fun of other people becomes a "sport" for these families. It's very hurtful to others, and for people who judge others, they do so because they have an insecure sense of themselves. Bringing this to the client's attention and helping them to become more sensitive and open-minded about other people will be an important part of recovery from codependency. For many, they don't realize that what they are doing is hurtful to others. And many children growing up in this environment begin to believe that if their family is critical of others, their family must be critical of them as well. So their self-esteem suffers.

Thus, self-righteousness is born from this judgmentalism. Those who have a self-righteous attitude look down on other people. They think of themselves above reproach and their way of living is right, and other's way of living is wrong. Self-righteousness is a tough issue to break down because it has been the way the individual identifies who they are. And if they change that view, then who are they? How do they ultimately fit into their family system? Breaking through this attitude may take some time. Be patient.

Spirituality/Sense of Self

I. LOSS OF SOUL/LOSS OF SELF

Codependents are prone to "lose themselves." In other words, they do not function authentically. Their focus is solely directed on other people and they end up not knowing who they are, what they want, or what they believe. I've seen this in both men and women. Many people can get stuck here and what I'll typically hear from my clients include, "I don't know what I want," "I feel like I've lost myself," and "I've given so much to everyone else I have nothing left." You'll hear this loss of self by people who have been selfless, probably for most of their lives. It's a huge loss and one in which the client needs to reclaim.

SPIRITUALITY/ SENSE OF SELF

1. Loss of Soul/Loss of Self
2. Spiritually Disconnected

I define the soul as the essence of who we are. Our soul involves our heart, our desires, and our beliefs, and includes our personality and the individual God intended for us to be.

I have seen people who are so unsure about who they are that they become "chameleons." As I discussed in Chapter 2, what this means is that they take on some of the personality traits of the person with whom they are interacting. So if someone is vivacious and outgoing and they are interacting with someone who is subdued and more introverted, the codependent person will act more subdued and introverted rather than their true self. Their "self" gets lost. Their soul gets lost.

2. SPIRITUALLY DISCONNECTED

Spiritually, many codependents get disconnected from God. Or they may have come from families who were not spiritually-minded. Unfortunately, if they've had people in their lives who have failed them or let them down in some way, the belief is that God will do the same. So a close, spiritual relationship is not something they pursue.

I've met people who are so filled with shame, they don't believe God can accept them, much less love them. This too, leads to isolation and shamefulness along with feeling unworthy of God's love.

Many codependents are capable and competent in many areas of their lives, and because they do take care of many things so well, they begin to trust in themselves only. Their trust in their own abilities alleviates their need for God. Also, their focus on others is much like an addiction and thus other important relationships slip away...even their relationship with God.

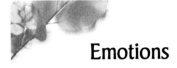

Emotions

I. FEAR OF ABANDONMENT/FEAR OF INTIMACY

Codependents fear abandonment and are also overwhelmed by intimacy (Timmens, pg. 19). These qualities develop in early childhood because they have had family members "leave" for a variety of reasons, such as death, emotional disconnection, and physically leaving the family. Their anxiety and fear become so high, they will do whatever it takes to keep connected to their dysfunctional family member. So you will see clients staying in unhealthy and even abusive relationships even when they know it's destructive.

> **EMOTIONS**
>
> 1. Fear of Abandonment/Fear of Intimacy
> 2. Fear of Conflict
> 3. Shame/Guilt
> 4. Powerlessness
> 5. Unaware of Emotions/Emotions Out of Control

Many clients have lost loved ones and never felt as though they had any emotional connection with those important people. When parents are unavailable emotionally, it's a loss for the child. This loss develops into major adult anxiety and fear that others will "leave" them.

In contrast, codependents are also afraid of intimacy, because they have had unhealthy people infiltrate their boundaries due to emotional problems. These relationships were "too close" and they build a protective wall to keep others at a distance emotionally. As you can imagine, adult relationships suffer and the couple will struggle with closeness.

2. FEAR OF CONFLICT

Codependents are terrified of conflict. When conflict arises, they may feel that they haven't done their job keeping things "perfect" or "under control." Shame comes over them and it's so uncomfortable to feel the shame, it's better to avoid the conflict, anger and pain at all costs.

It's ironic, then, that people with codependency may stir up problems if things in their life are too calm, only to be frightened by the conflict that evolves. When people avoid conflict, they ultimately lose their option to discuss things with their loved ones and they learn to avoid certain topics. Their communication becomes nonexistent and unhealthy and they have trouble communicating directly with anyone in their life.

Often, I've seen an enormous amount of anxiety in these people as well. They may have experienced an array of abuse and any little bit of conflict can trigger them into their fear. I've also worked with people who fear conflict because they never saw people in their lives fight, get angry, or maybe not seen parents argue and make up. So conflict is scary for them.

3. SHAME/GUILT

People living in these unhealthy situations carry a lot of shame. They feel embarrassed about themselves and about their situation. Shame can be described as a wave that comes over them washing them with a feeling that they are no good. They feel defective. It's not just that they do things wrong, they ARE wrong. Their sense of self is devalued and does not matter.

I believe guilt, on the other hand, can be an important emotion and can help people stay on the right path. When someone feels guilt, for example, they realize the need to change their course or give an apology to someone they have hurt. That's a good thing. But an over-abundance of guilt keeps clients stuck. Both shame and guilt are difficult to heal from because the healing must come from a deep core belief about oneself. People are left feeling guilt and shame their entire lives because they're unwilling to dig down deep and address their very painful emotions.

Self-care: I feel guilty when I do...I feel guilty when I don't.

4. POWERLESSNESS

Many codependents actually feel powerless, and their need for control is a failed attempt at achieving this desired goal of power. Powerlessness leads to feelings of failure and that of being a victim, which often creates a lonely place from which the individual lives. It will be important for therapists to help the client realize the only power and control they have is control of themselves. Many people understand this intellectually, but because of pain in their past, they have difficulty "letting go" of these controlling behaviors. The negative beliefs about themselves and the false sense of control they believe they have, is exactly what we need to address.

5. UNAWARE OF EMOTIONS/EMOTIONS OUT OF CONTROL

Many codependent families had two extremes when it came to emotional responses. Some families never learned to identify their feelings and the codependent person learned to hide or "stuff" their emotions. Other families had reactions that were overflowing, abusive and ultimately out of control. Some children who expressed themselves emotionally may have been told to "Stop crying or I'll give you something to cry about!" Unhealthy emotional intimacy between children and parents and between husband and wife generally are either out of control or hidden in these families.

Healthy family systems manage their feelings well. Ideally, children and adults were taught to identify and to experience emotions in appropriate ways. For example, anger was not used abusively to punish the children. The children learned to manage anger in productive, respectful ways, like pounding pillows or journaling about their feelings. Love was freely expressed to one another and joy was a part of the fabric of the family and abounded all around them.

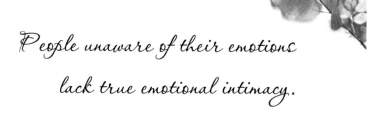

People unaware of their emotions lack true emotional intimacy.

I have had clients who made a decision in their childhood not to express anger like their father, as an example, because his emotions were out of control and abusive, and they felt their only recourse was to keep their own anger hidden and underground. They may have been scared of the anger that was expressed by their dad because it was violent. Unfortunately, what transpires is they didn't learn to express their anger appropriately in their marriage and other important adult relationships and it builds up over time until they finally explode. After these explosions, then guilt and remorse take over and they become ashamed of themselves for expressing their emotions so abruptly.

Another example of overflowing emotions involves sex addicts. Talking about sex and managing sexual feelings was not part of their conversation with their parents when they were young. They hadn't learned from older, wiser people in their lives how to express their sexuality in healthy ways. These poorly-informed people, then, become over-sexualized in their adult life because they didn't learn to manage their sexual feelings as an adolescent or teen.

I've also seen people and couples who saw little emotion shared between family members and they were unable to identify and express feelings in their adult relationships. Without these feelings expressed, children can have difficulty with attachment issues. They have not felt connected or loved by the adults in their life and then have difficulty connecting with their partners and children.

Poor or abusive emotional expression can wreak havoc on families and continue from generation to generation. Our work will take time and effort as we teach our clients how to identify emotions, what vocabulary to use to identify those feelings and then how to express the affect in appropriate ways.

IN SUMMARY: This is only a partial list of emotions that will come up in your counseling setting and you will need to address all of them. Identifying the emotions, expressing them and releasing them will bring healing.

It's obvious that codependency has many traits and not all codependent people have all the traits I have identified. But use this overview of characteristics as a way to identify codependency concerns for your clients. On the next page, I have included an assessment for codependency that is helpful to determine if it's a problem for your clients.

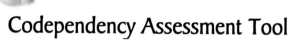

Codependency Assessment Tool

This is an exercise in curiosity not in self-criticism.

Codependency makes it difficult to see your own thoughts, feelings and actions clearly because your focus is primarily on others. In codependency, value comes from the opinions of others and safety comes from feeling needed. Be curious. The beginning of recovery is getting to know yourself more clearly. Take your time completing this.

1. My relationships often involve people who need my help or are somehow dependent on me.
2. When I can't help someone, I feel guilty and responsible for their upset feelings.
3. In the last year, significant others have resorted to arguing, begging or raising their voice to get me to stop trying to help them.
4. I spend a lot of time thinking through or projecting outcomes, trying to figure out what I can do to get the outcome I want.
5. It's difficult for me to receive praise or thanks from others.
6. I do not like to let myself get angry. When I do, I often lose control and feel ashamed.
7. It's difficult for me to say "No" or to ask for things that I need at home, at work, or with friends.
8. I often over-commit my time and measure my self-esteem by how much someone depends on me.
9. It is hard for me to have fun or relax; if I'm not productive, I feel worthless.
10. It's difficult to believe that someone could truly love me.
11. I am afraid of being hurt or abandoned if I allow myself to be loved.
12. I find it easy to criticize and blame others, although I don't like to admit it.
13. I seem to justify or make excuses for others' actions when they have hurt me.
14. When I know a relationship is about to end, I will stay in it until I can begin another relationship.
15. It is easy to make me feel guilty because I take responsibility for others and blame myself for their upset.
16. I am not sure what normal is.
17. I often take a stand in a relationship and then go back on what I said if it causes tension.
18. I am not aware of what I want. I ask others what _they_ want.
19. I tend to be sick a lot. I can't seem to fight off infection, but it doesn't stop me.
20. There never seems to be enough time to do things I enjoy.

The Journey of Recovery: The New Testament

Codependency Assessment Scoring

If you answered "Yes" to more than
6 questions, then codependency
is clearly part of your relationships.

You are known to be helpful,
self-sacrificing, hard-working,
trustworthy and self-sufficient.

What turns these strengths into
codependency is when you
"need to be needed" in order
to believe you have any value.

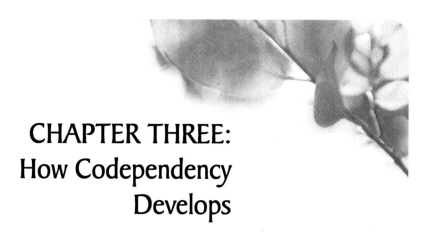

CHAPTER THREE:
How Codependency
Develops

Codependency develops in early childhood. As children grow and learn to interact in their environment, they are impacted by the healthiness of their family system which includes immediate family and extended family i.e., siblings, parents, grandparents, aunts and uncles, cousins, and earlier members who came before them. Genetic issues, emotional health or mental health problems can get passed from one generation to the next.

Some families with little to no emotional expression look very healthy on the outside as the members succeed in life; however, they lack awareness of feelings and how to share those emotions with others which causes relationships that are cold, sterile, and disconnected. This will perpetuate intimacy problems into their adulthood. The children are starved for healthy touch, emotional connection and understanding feelings. They acquire little information about relationships and other life lessons. These issues become so engrained in their character that in order to "redo" or adjust their thoughts, feelings and beliefs, it will first take awareness of the difficulties and then determination and stamina to learn new strategies.

When the family has had chronic mental or physical health problems, children can experience extremes from abuse to neglect. If the family lacks structure, clients come into the therapy office feeling disconnected, scattered and confused. They may have been left alone when they were too young to care for themselves or their siblings. Often, if the older child has had to care for the younger kids, the care-giving child becomes more and more resentful. Too many young children have more responsibility than they can handle. When they lack skills for this responsibility, they learn they are incompetent early in life and that core belief of "I'm not good enough" continues into their adulthood. Also, many have experienced extreme neglect and the children lacked healthy touch, as well as the basic needs of food, shelter, clothing, medical/dental care, etc. Fear of abandonment permeates their psyche and, as adults, they will stay in unhealthy, abusive relationships too long.

Codependency flourishes in families who have difficulty with emotional expression, chronic mental or physical problems, neglect, abuse and addiction.

Abuse can be rampant in all these unhealthy families. Boundaries are continually violated and children don't learn how to say "No," because no one taught them it's OK to say that if someone is hurting or abusing them. This is a set-up for future abuse and they stay stuck. They learn to think they are worthless and there will be a need to address this worthlessness in therapy in order to make positive strides in life. The power of the negative beliefs is astounding and many people live their entire life feeling "Not good enough."

Addictive families don't know how to regulate their emotions and are certainly not in any position to focus on their children's issues. Their addiction takes priority and the children have had to learn life skills on their own. Codependents must learn how to make decisions, manage relationships, and regulate emotions without the wisdom of a parent or adult caregiver. When they learn these strategies alone at an early age, their emotional regulation is juvenile and immature. Often boundaries are lacking in these families along with physical, emotional, sexual and spiritual abuse. The families have a self-righteous attitude toward others and view the world in black and white, right or wrong and good or bad. Individuals in these families may teach certain spiritual truths but don't live those truths. So, children get a double message and it makes for a very confusing upbringing and poor emotional intimacy, to say the least.

When children don't have a nurturing environment and their parents are MIA (missing in action) for whatever reason, they may have endured yelling, criticism, profanity, mind-games, emotional and physical incest, physical abuse (hitting, slapping, pushing, witnessing others being abused), lack of healthy sexual discussion, touching inappropriately, teasing about bodies, sarcasm, no privacy, sexual experimentation with older kids and adults, and exposure to pornography and sexual humor. Unfortunately immature and ineffective coping strategies learned in their early years stay with the children for a lifetime unless there is some kind of counseling intervention. Teaching is of utmost importance in the counseling they receive as the new, healthy relationship skills are learned and practiced. It always surprises me the lack of information codependents possess and how excited they are when they begin learning new life skills and when they embrace new positive beliefs about themselves.

Everyone experiences pain from others and many of those hurts are processed normally and we can "get over" that pain. But those deeper hurts can linger. For example, if a client has unmet needs for love and acceptance, they can become numb, unfeeling, or the other extreme: rage-filled. These feelings and extremes can drive people with codependency to please others and seek their approval. Rather than have a drive to please oneself, the individual becomes unknowingly (and sometimes knowingly) focused on pleasing other people. And of course there is no control in that situation either. The path they are following is focused on others and not on themselves.

Neglect contributes to kids feeling uncertain of themselves.

In my research I've found many family characteristics that are common in this disorder (see the next page). I have compiled a list of family characteristics from the many codependency books I've read. What I notice with this list is that the characteristics are the extreme. In other words, codependency develops because of too much of something or too little of something. So as therapists, we need to help our clients find the balance in their lives, as well as help them to balance their thoughts, feelings and behaviors.

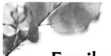

Family Codependency Characteristics

- Alcoholism
- Other Addictions
- Workaholism
- Divorce
- Eating Disorders
- Sexual Disorders
- Absent Father
- Absent Mother
- Neglect
- Need to Please
- Spiritual Rigidity

- Verbal Abuse
- Emotional Abuse
- Physical Abuse
- Sexual Abuse
- Domineering Father/Passive Mother
- Domineering Mother/Passive Father
- Attachment/Relationships Issues

Another important consideration for how codependency develops includes the health of the early attachment style for the child. Attachment is not a new concept. It's a helpful description to understand how children learn to relate to others. Many people who have developed codependent strategies have learned unhealthy attachment styles and have learned to bond to caregivers in dysfunctional ways. When children have not attached well in their first years of life, future relationships will be negatively impacted. Codependent adults will have difficulty with emotional intimacy in their marriage and with their children by being "needy" and suffocating, or they will be detached and aloof. As with other codependency characteristics, these are the extremes.

Ideally children should have "secure" attachment styles. When parents are tuned-in to their child and the child's emotional and physical needs are met, the child feels secure in themselves and can have close, intimate relationships without an immense amount of anxiety and fear. These families typically are healthy emotionally and the "attuned interplay throughout childhood, where the emotional needs of the child are met, becomes the foundation for a secure sense of self and successful future relationships." (Shapiro, pg. 102)

When parents are tuned-in to their kids, secure attachments are made.

According to Shapiro's research, insecure attachment style occurs about 35% of the time. When children have had poor connection with their parents, or they have experienced trauma or abuse, they may show uncomfortable feelings with closeness and expressions of love and other strong emotions. You can understand that alcoholic parents or chronic mental or physical illness in the primary caregiver can disrupt this connection. When you have these problems in the family, the parent may be unable to provide the connection with their child. Their focus becomes their own issues rather than the needs of the child.

When there is an insecure attachment style, children grow up feeling they are unloved or unlovable, and unworthy. They grow up learning to keep their emotions to themselves because when they shared emotions or desires in their unhealthy families their needs were not met and they learned to keep their emotions bottled up. They may have seen parents pull away from them and close off emotions. Parents with this attachment style may avoid kissing or touching their children because it's just too uncomfortable for them to do so.

In the dismissive attachment style, children's physical needs are met, but their emotional needs are neglected or "dismissed." They don't intend to hurt their children; they are just doing what they learned as children from their parents. Their response becomes an automatic one that offers little warmth and connection. We can see this attachment style in people who we may view as "cold," or hard-hearted. Many couples come in to our offices with one of the partners having trouble being emotionally or physically intimate with their partner. This attachment style has life-long repercussions.

Preoccupied attachment is another insecure attachment style where the parents have their own issues and struggles that preoccupy them from providing healthy attachment. They may have a lot of anger and anxiety and when their own triggers happen, they have difficulty separating emotionally from their issues to take care of the children. The children's' needs can be a trigger for them. And we can see this in families where one parent or the other has chronic health issues, chronic mental health issues, or drug and alcohol problems.

Attachment problems contribute to codependency.

The family can also look like a narcissistic family system. The children are not as important as, or even the focus of, the parent or caregiver. Children begin to feel unimportant, not heard and understood, and will ultimately have difficulty with other relationships. Again, codependency develops from this background and as adults, the individual is insecure, clingy, anxious, demanding and overly dependent on others.

For many adults who have trauma in their history, the insecure attachment style that affects their children is called disorganized attachment. Children with these issues are fearful and can be traumatized because of their parents' angry outbursts, abuse, and anxious behaviors. As Shapiro explains, "The very person to whom they want to run to for comfort is at the same time the source of their anxiety." (pg. 103) As the children get older they can be demanding, controlling and throwing tantrums if they don't get what they want. Other children with this history can be depressed and "look frozen." (pg. 104)

Again, codependency can develop from this attachment style. As children become adults, they may have learned to be controlling in their environment and in their relationships due to the anxiety they felt as young children. They can become hyper-vigilant and fearful of many, many things that can exasperate partners and children who have loved ones like this.

We do know, however, that these dysfunctional attachment styles, along with the codependency that develops, can be reversed by being in a relationship with loving people. If the child has had a few loving role models like a teacher, neighbor, coach, or friend their attachment issues may be lessened. Also, healing the wounds of their past can bring relief, as well as lower anxiety and depression, along with hope for a more satisfying future. New ways of managing emotions, behaviors and relationships can be learned. Working through the difficult issues is critical in order for healing and this book, I'm hoping, will be a helpful tool for therapists to make a great difference in their clients' lives.

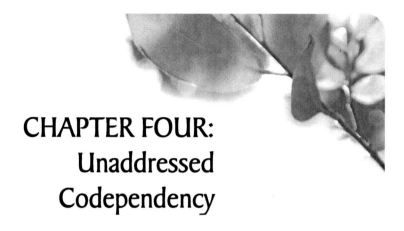

CHAPTER FOUR:
Unaddressed
Codependency

When codependency goes unaddressed, it can result in very serious health issues. Codependents may have learned poor coping strategies to deal with their struggles and we need to understand what kinds of coping mechanisms they have learned and discuss healthier options for them. It's important as well to assess for other emotional and mental health concerns because we know that unhealthy family dynamics can lead to other mental health conditions.

For example, many codependent people have turned to alcoholism or other addictions to manage their emotions. For others, their stress levels are so high and they feel so overwhelmed with responsibility that they have developed health issues such as ulcers, headaches, asthma, digestive problems, high blood pressure, etc. And due to the unhealthiness of addictive families, you will most likely see high anxiety and depression levels, panic disorders, and even PTSD. Also be very careful and aware of suicidal ideation. People with codependency can feel so overwhelmed and have such difficulty managing their world, that suicide may look like an attractive way to escape their pain.

Struggles that arise for the individual can look somewhat different in everyone, but as you take a closer look at the individual and family system, you will find commonalities. These are some of the presenting problems that I've seen come into my counseling office:

- A concern or dissatisfaction with their marriage and/or other relationships.
- Feeling unhappy, fearful, depressed, anxious, and may have suicidal thinking and panic attacks.
- Difficulty focusing on themselves. They are overly focused on the behaviors of the other person(s) and have trouble believing they can't change them. They might intellectually and cognitively know that, but they have great difficulty with redirecting their focus and changing the belief that they can "help" that loved one.
- Critical of themselves, their partners or family members, and life in general.
- Frustration with lack of control of other's behaviors.
- Work issues, feeling unhappy at work, upset about a co-worker and difficulty getting along with others.
- Lack of balance in their lives and exhibiting high anxiety, depression and have great feelings of being overwhelmed.
- Exhaustion because they've tried for years to take care of or control others and have felt frustrated and discouraged.
- Powerlessness. They may have had some luck feeling in control of others or their life, but at some point they don't feel that others are listening to them or doing what they "should" be doing any longer. This word "should" is a common word in their vocabulary.
- "Black and white" thinking and believing people should or shouldn't do things, things are right or wrong, good or bad, horrible or wonderful. Again, because of their black and white mentality and actions, they may struggle with relationships due to the skewed perspective they hold on to.
- "Bound and tormented by the way things were in their dysfunctional family of origin," according to Hemfelt, Minirth and Meier. (pg. 21) These

individuals have strong feelings and reactions to their family and loved ones from their past.

- Moods and feelings out of control. Anger can be explosive, depression is deep, and other emotions over the top.

- Defensiveness and protective of themselves and their loved ones as a way to keep from getting hurt.

- Lives become destructive in that they don't know how to take care of themselves. They may have very little support, may also punish themselves with criticism, shame, or have behaviors such as alcoholism, eating disorders, etc. from the inability to cope well.

- Does not feel authentic. They may feel a certain way, but act another. They give up themselves and their desires for others' needs or demands.

- Don't know who they are, what they like or don't like, and live contradictory to their values.

- Confused about what they want or need. They are unfamiliar with the concept of having needs because their lives may have been so focused on other's needs.

- Exhibit passive-aggressive behaviors and yet tell people they are not mad, but may retaliate against someone with sarcasm or abuse.

- Feel self-righteous in that they've lived life in the "right" way and others have not, so they criticize others and/or feel they are above them.

- Become perfectionistic to cover up their lack of self-esteem, relationship issues and unhealthy behaviors.

- Feeling stuck in their situation and don't know what to do to make change happen.

- Continues to protect, be angry with, and cover up for the other person -- nothing changes, except the codependent person may become more exhausted and frustrated that they can't control them.

- Unhealthy mistaken beliefs. For example, they may believe it's up to them to save the other person from themselves. They also may believe all relationships are like theirs, that it's up to them to care for others, or that other people are not capable of taking care of themselves, etc.

- Physically, emotionally, psychologically, and spiritually sick due to neglect and other health issues. They may have chronic health issues, chronic pain, and other physical symptoms. Also, if feelings are not expressed, the individual may become physically sick or mentally sick because of unresolved issues and emotions "stuffed" for many years.

- Feel angry towards God, disconnected or believe they are being punished by God. They are upset because God has not intervened in a positive way or answered their prayers. Because the individual is so focused on others, their relationship with God becomes neglected. They have learned to rely on themselves, so there is no need for God.

- Difficulty understanding clear and healthy boundaries. They have had little experience or education about what healthy boundaries look like and they continue to intrude in other peoples' lives by giving advice, making recommendations for how to live life, and even demand that other people do things their way, which can include sexual demands as well.

- Feel or present like a "victim," where they are not at fault and that what has happened hasn't been because of them but because of what others have done. This victim mentality can be a stubborn trait to change because their need to stay in the victim role is necessary to define for themselves who they are.

- Feel or present like a "martyr," where they explain they have done so much sacrificing for others to the detriment of themselves. Breaking away from this role can be difficult because, much like the victim role, it defines them and without that definition of themselves, who are they?

- Great need to be accepted. They may want to get close or impress the therapist, so be careful about the client/therapist boundaries. Their kindness can be a slippery slope for therapists especially if the therapist has some codependency issues themselves.

Be sure to consider codependency as one of the issues if these presenting problems come into your office (see the list on the next page). Let the client know that deciding to seek counseling is a great step in recovery. First, identifying the disorder becomes a relief for many because they are miserable but don't understand why. And learning new strategies to strengthen their own self esteem and their relationships can be a welcome change.

Presenting Issues Coming into the Office

- Marital or relationship problems
- Anxiety, worry, fearful, suicidal
- Hyper-focus on others
- Critical of self
- Frustration with lack of control of others
- Work issues
- Lack of balance in life
- Exhaustion, abuse & feeling taken advantage of
- Powerlessness
- Black & white thinking
- Dysfunctional family-of-origin
- Inability to manage affect
- Defensiveness
- Destructive lives
- Lacks authenticity
- Variety of abuse issues
- Doesn't know self
- Confusion about a variety of things
- Destructive lives
- Passive-aggressive
- Self-righteous
- Perfectionism
- Stuck
- Protective of loved ones
- Unhealthy mistaken beliefs
- Physically, emotionally, spiritually sick
- Feel punished, angry & disconnected from God
- Unhealthy/unclear boundaries
- Victim
- Martyr
- Great need for acceptance

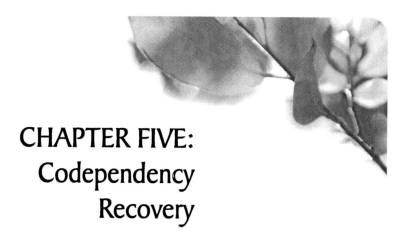

CHAPTER FIVE:
Codependency
Recovery

On page 65 is a quick overview of the topics you will be addressing in codependency recovery. Take your time and remember to walk alongside your clients, not pushing or moving too quickly, but also not staying stuck in one or two areas. It's a fine balance, but it can be done.

Codependency is a very deep-rooted issue to recover from and it is very difficult to make the changes from codependency to healthy living in a short amount of time. It can take years to recover from this problem due to the varied issues that need to be addressed and also due to the longevity of the problem in many people's lives...for some people it's been a lifetime of unhealthy living.

Treatment for codependency is definitely not linear. Untangling issues and disorders for codependency is messy work. We may help them address one area of their life, such as teaching boundaries, then move to assertiveness training, and on to helping them understand their family system, then identify feelings, and address accepting the issue/problem and back again to assertiveness training. It's much like a maze, in and out, up and down, back and forth. Are you ready for the ride?

All of these issues listed on the next page need to be addressed throughout the process of counseling for codependency. Also, as with any client, a thorough understanding of issues and concerns is important; however, remember that listening is one of the most important therapy approaches you can offer someone with codependency.

Therapy Strategies to
Treat Codependency

Step 1: **Therapists Assess Yourselves**

Step 2: **Psychology 101**
- Do a Thorough Intake
- Build Rapport
- Listen Carefully
- Set Goals
- Be Patient with the Client
- Provide Love & Belonging/ Unconditional Positive Regard

Step 3: **Safety, Support & Growth**
- Identify Safe People
- Build Support
- Identify & Express Emotions
- Teach Self-Care
- Detach with Love

Step 4: **Codependent Treatment Difficulties**
- Redirect the Client's Focus on Others
- Move Clients from Denial to Awareness
- Deal with Resistance
- Deal with Control Issues

Step 5: **Healing From the Ground Up**
- Address Family-of-Origin Issues
- Build Self-Esteem
- Identify and Set Healthy Boundaries
- Address Body Responses
- Address Trauma
- Discuss Spiritual Renewal

Step 1: Therapists Assess Yourselves

Are you codependent? Many therapists are. So it's important that we all assess ourselves for the issue of codependency. Maybe you find yourself siding with one spouse or the other in the counseling setting. Maybe you take on the feelings of your clients and hurt because they hurt or you're angry because they are angry. These can be codependent behaviors.

Many codependent people get into the helping profession because it comes very naturally for them to help others. We feel compassionate toward others and love the fact that people like our advice and suggestions. Before I started in this field, I felt as though I did counseling for some of my family and friends. It came naturally for me. But was it healthy? Was I offering my advice when I was not asked for my advice? Was I simply taking on their problems and trying to fix those problems when they really weren't mine to fix?

Codependency is a very insidious problem and we may say to ourselves "I'm only trying to help." But in fact, we're intruding on others. Ask yourself, did this individual ask for my input? Did they want to be "fixed?" As we work with clients, we can easily get caught up in their "story" or their chaos.

Be careful not to get too invested in your clients and/or work harder than they are. If you are working harder, then that means you're too invested. If you're feeling frustrated and angry that the client is not making changes or progressing in their therapy, step back and look at your own issues. Or, if you're thinking about your clients when you're not at work and have difficulty letting go of the thoughts and concerns about a client, you may be too involved. If you can't get away from thinking or worrying or trying to fix your client, assess your involvement, consider codependency as a problem for you and get some outside support.

HOW CAN WE HELP? As a new therapist, I had a young girl who was struggling with her relationships with her parents. Mom and dad were divorced. Mom was actively using illegal drugs and bringing strange people into their home. Dad was a drug dealer and had little time for this young girl. I began to feel very concerned for her safety. I did call Child Protection to see if there was anything I needed to report, but unfortunately, there was no abuse to report. It was one of only a couple clients I've had where I wanted to step in and take her home with me and protect her and show her the love she deserved. I was too involved and my codependency was showing itself.

If you find yourself in this position, reach out to a colleague or someone who understands codependency and learn some strategies to detach. I found myself thinking about my young client often and it was distracting to my other personal relationships. I worried about her, prayed for her safety, but it got in the way of being emotionally present for my family. What I did do, however, was plan a self-defense class for girls her age and invited her to be a part of that class. It felt good to help by offering her ideas on how to protect herself, providing emotional support for her through the school year, and I encouraged her to ask for help from school or other "safe" people in her life if she needed it.

So get help for yourself first and take care of your own issues before treating others. Too many of us have grown up in chemically-addicted or dysfunctional homes and have many of the characteristics of codependency. Again, your hearts are in the right place and we want to help others, but do your own work first and you will be able to provide the best counseling care for your clients.

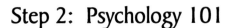

Step 2: Psychology 101

- ## DO A THOROUGH INTAKE

    As new clients come in to your office it's important to assess for trauma, addiction and neglect. A thorough assessment will identify many issues right away. Good questions narrow down the issues pretty clearly and you can ask the client to elaborate on those areas that need attention.

    Be sure to assess your clients for the typical things like, anxiety, depression, other mental health diagnoses, abuse, neglect, their own chemical or relationship dependencies, but also keep tuned in to see if there is any Post-Traumatic Stress Disorder (PTSD). Due to the dysfunction many codependents live with, they may have experienced very traumatic upbringings and may have some PTSD symptoms. Many addictive homes have exhibited unhealthy coping strategies and in these toxic environments, unfortunately, many parents and caregivers have used their codependent children to meet their needs. This includes emotional needs, sexual needs, physical and psychological needs.

    If your client has experienced any kind of abuse, be sure you are trained to work with trauma or PTSD. If you are not trained in these areas, it's best to refer your clients to another therapist who is trained in working with trauma or work collaboratively with a trauma therapist.

    If your client is facing issues that may get in the way of successful counseling, consider what Cermak recommends. He encourages that the therapist consider these five factors before starting therapy:

✓ Is the client using drugs and/or alcohol, or any mood altering medication?

✓ Is the home environment conducive to recovery?

✓ Have you assessed for PTSD?

✓ Is group therapy a good option for this client?

✓ What stage of recovery is the client in?

HOW CAN WE HELP? If you find your client is using drugs or alcohol to cope, ideally it's better to address the chemical abuse first. It's important for the client to be able to tolerate strong feelings without a mood altering affect. Helping the client find a place to get treatment for their chemical use will be important. And consider that codependency may be an issue as many people struggling with addictions are also codependent.

However, we know that not all clients are receptive to getting that help first. They don't always believe they are chemically addicted. I struggle with this particular approach because I have worked with clients who are using alcohol as a coping strategy. I have seen progress in spite of their chemical use. In the safety of the counseling setting, after trust has built, and as the client begins to address some of the pain of their codependency and their abuse, then we can talk more about getting help for their chemical abuse. However, I believe the process can take longer if they continue their unhealthy coping strategies, whatever they may be.

Much like assessing for chemical or drug abuse, it will be important to know if there are other mental health issues that need attention before working on the codependency issues. So remember to do a thorough assessment and intake to address other pressing needs that warrant attention before addressing the codependency issues.

- **BUILD RAPPORT**

As you're going through their intake information, you will want to be aware of the important step of building rapport. Clients need to feel safe and trust that you have their best interest at heart.

People with codependency either trust too much or don't trust enough. For those individuals who have had trauma, or any wounding experiences, they can be the client that comes in the door and loves you to death or they can be the client that is very difficult to connect with. Building rapport is very important and to you it may seem like an easy part of our job, but it can definitely be challenging.

What I do for new clients coming in to see me is to offer a free 30-minute consultation. I want to have them come into my office and see the surroundings, feel the calmness and comfort my office provides, and I take time to connect with that client. Those first 30-minutes can be crucial in starting to build rapport and connecting so the client will come back for future sessions as well as feel safe in this first consult. They also need to feel that you are skilled enough to help them, so be sure and let them know what training you've had and what skills you possess.

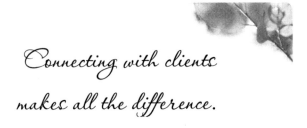

Connecting with clients makes all the difference.

My goal in this first encounter is to make them comfortable and show them that they are cared about and accepted no matter what issues they bring into my office. I encourage them and offer hope no matter what the situation. I also offer ideas of what we can do together to make their life work better for them.

HOW CAN WE HELP? When I meet with new clients I will spend a little time telling them who I am. I'll talk about my licensing, the training I've taken, the type of therapy I do, for example, EMDR (Eye Movement Desensitization and Reprocessing), and how I interact with my clients (I offer ideas, psycho-education, etc). I believe it's important for them to know who they are talking to and answer questions they may have about me.

As you know, there are some clients who don't really care who you are. They just dive right in and start to tell you their story. So you may have to go with the flow, but eventually, it's important to help them understand who you are.

With most clients I do share with them that I grew up in an alcoholic home and that codependency was an issue I struggled with and am skilled at, along with other issues like anxiety, depression, abuse and trauma. I will talk about how important counseling was for me in my healing journey.

My experience has shown me that some people have difficulty connecting because of their trauma, PTSD, and other struggles where their trust has been broken. If their trust issues get in the way, take your time and know that building rapport is paramount before getting too far into their issues.

- **LISTEN CAREFULLY**
I know, I know, this is a no brainer, but it's an important step. As you build rapport you will be listening intently and you will also be listening for important clues into the issues of codependency. Remember, listening is very therapeutic for clients, especially those presenting with codependency

issues because being heard and understood by people in their life may not have happened.

I believe individuals need time to purge their thoughts and feelings in the beginning stages of counseling. Don't try to move the client too quickly through this first phase of therapy. Be cognizant to pace yourself and the client.

"Having someone listen to me made my situation more bearable."

With addiction being such a selfish issue, many people with codependency have had few people, if any, who have really listened to them or cared about what they thought, felt and believed. So being available as a great listener can offer an enormous amount of support and encouragement. For the first time, they may realize that no one has really had much interest in them. It will probably be very uncomfortable for them, as well, to be the focus of the session, but it's exactly what they need.

"For the first time my counselor really listened to me. She looked me in the eyes and seemed very interested in what I had to say. Of course my trust was not great when I started counseling and I struggled with negative self-talk in my head saying it was just her job to listen. She was getting paid to listen. She doesn't really care. But it was so helpful and I felt such relief after just one session. Having someone hear me and understand my situation was so calming for my fears and anxiety and for the first time I felt as if I'm important. I couldn't wait for my next session.

It was wonderful." This from a client who was just starting the counseling process and realizing she was dealing with codependency issues.

HOW CAN WE HELP? When I first meet the client, I am genuinely interested to hear their story. I stay focused, pay attention to what they are telling me, and I'm also listening for loss; loss of self, loss of dreams, loss of soul. As I listen to them, I'm formulating a plan to help treat the issue of codependency. It's critical for the client to feel safe and when they do, they will be more open and willing to go emotionally deeper and reach healing.

What the client thinks and feels matters, but often, with codependency, they have no sense of any importance about their thoughts and feelings especially if they tend to think of others ahead of themselves. Listening with compassion is a great skill and is very therapeutic in and of itself. Carl Rogers knew this and you know it, too, so don't minimize this integral step.

- **SET GOALS**
  At the first intake session I'm always thinking about goals. What specifically does the client want to accomplish? I then collaborate with them to formulate a plan, combining the client's ideas along with what I think would be helpful for their recovery. Some clients will have very specific ideas and others will not know what they want. As therapists, that's our job to help give them direction and offer hope along with specific treatment options.

With a plan we can determine if changes are happening. I have found that many clients are unaware of what changes they have made or they are unaware of what interventions have been helpful. These evolutions can be so subtle that it will be important to identify for the client where they have grown.

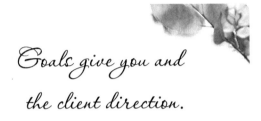

Goals give you and the client direction.

Being skilled to treat codependency is imperative and when the client knows that you have the skills to treat their issues, they will experience relief. Use ideas from this book to address the nuances that go along with this issue.

HOW CAN WE HELP? Ideally, planning the therapy goals is important in the first session; however, some clients may not be able to accomplish this until several sessions in. Some clients come with a lot to say and they need that time to purge their thoughts and feelings, and many need time to tell their story. The telling of their history relieves much anxiety and I encourage you to allow them that time. Don't worry if you don't set a plan until the second or third session. One initial goal I try to get to the first session is self-care. Most clients with codependency come in exhausted and overwhelmed and know little about taking care of themselves.

Part of our assessment for codependency will be looking to see if there are any Family Codependency Characteristics (see page 53). As you review this list, you can help identify what other goals can be set. And if we determine together that there are codependency issues, I will let them know about the steps I have outlined here so they know I can help them. I go over the Therapy Strategies for Codependency on page 65 and review this with them to explain the process. It's important to give them hope that change can happen and they don't have to do it alone.

I also make a point of checking in on the goals periodically throughout our process, for example, six weeks down the road. This helps the client understand what progress they've made. I also affirm for them all along the way the things they are doing well, such as identifying ways in which they've been courageous, or the fact that they've done a great job with setting boundaries as well as any other signs of recovery. They love hearing this and it's also nice for the therapist to know what interventions were helpful.

• BE PATIENT WITH THE CLIENT

Patience is an important quality for therapists working with codependency. This issue is so woven into the fabric of who our clients are, there will be issues we have to break through: for example, denial, unhealthy behaviors and faulty beliefs, and control issues. You may feel as though your therapy is not helping the client. The clients may be stuck, which causes us frustration. I'm outlining for you a couple of ways you will be challenged when you work with this issue.

✓ **YOUR FRUSTRATION:** Working with codependency can be frustrating and tedious, so as therapists you will be challenged with your own patience. People with codependency are disengaged from their own issues and have difficulty focusing on themselves. Their focus is on others and you may find that they know more about their loved ones than themselves. For some, it may be the first time someone has asked them "How are you?" They may have difficulty answering that question or they may talk incessantly. Keeping them focused can be very challenging.

I have found "peer-vision" helpful while working with someone with codependency. Peervision is a way to consult with other therapists and discuss my frustration and to get another perspective. I believe it's helpful for all the counseling we do even years after getting licensed. It helps us stay focused and encourages us to look at our own issues.

✓ **YOUR IMPATIENCE:** Impatience can be a struggle for some therapists. Just a reminder, be gentle with yourself if you're feeling frustrated, angry, or hopelessly stuck. Just when you think your client is not making progress, they come in the next session reporting changes they've made, behaviors they've tried, and successes they've had. It may be important, too, for you to have support and have a support network of peers with whom you can consult. What triggers are happening for you as you work with this challenging issue? This is a good question to ask yourself.

- **PROVIDE LOVE & BELONGING/
  UNCONDITIONAL POSITIVE REGARD**
  I believe we get into the counseling world as therapists because we care about people. And providing love and belonging and unconditional positive regard probably comes naturally for many of us. However, you may have clients who come to you that you're not real fond of. What I've found is that as I've gotten to know the client better, I realize what part of love and acceptance they have missed growing up. Notice what part of belonging was neglected in their world? Once I understand this, I can learn to appreciate who they are and what struggles they have faced.

✓ **FIRST PHONE CALL:** A first step to provide love and belonging starts at the first phone call. We know that most clients are very nervous about calling us to begin with and if they have someone who is cold and impatient on the other line, the client will feel that. So expressing care and concern from the start will make a big difference for your clients.

✓ **WARM ATMOSPHERE**: It's also important to have an atmosphere of safety, calmness, acceptance and compassion, which we hope to provide for our clients. We want to offer them the sense of belonging and feeling loved or cared about. Simply being ready for the client, being on time, and genuinely glad to see them helps the client feel as though they are important. We offer beverages so clients feel welcome. That cup of tea may be just the thing for someone who is working on tough issues.

✓ **THE SEVEN DESIRES**: As therapists we understand that many of our clients have desires and needs that were unmet. We can help meet some of those longings by bringing understanding and comfort to our clients. I have found Dr. Mark and Debbie Laaser's book, *The Seven Desires*, a helpful tool to address the important desires of us all. Be aware of these as you work with codependency.

DESIRE 1: To Be Heard & Understood

Being listened to gives us a feeling of worth and that what we have to say is important enough to have others listen. I remember my first counseling session and I left that office overwhelmed with gratitude at being listened to, as I hadn't realized until then that I had missed this growing up. Laaser's book suggests, "If you had a childhood in which people talked to you--or worse, at you--but never really listened, you may have given up on talking...Sometimes our desire to be heard literally causes us to speak differently! When we want to communicate something important and feel we are not being heard, we might raise our voice, thinking that if we talk louder, maybe we will finally be heard. Alternately, if we want to be heard, sometimes we might say something more slowly...or we repeat ourselves, slowly." (Laaser, pg. 18, 19)

Notice how your clients are presenting themselves. Some have much to say and it's difficult to get a word in edgewise. Others will be difficult to talk with as they are tentative and hold back as well as have difficulty expressing their thoughts and feelings. For example, in my practice, when I have clients who are talking so quickly and without pause, I know that this client needs to be listened to. In fact, for the first couple of sessions, I will let them have the floor. I want them to feel heard and feel compassion from someone who knows how important it is to have a voice.

THE SEVEN DESIRES

1. To be heard & understood
2. To be affirmed
3. To be blessed
4. To be safe
5. To be touched
6. To be chosen
7. To be included

Likewise, I have also had clients who have said very little. Talking for them has been fruitless, so they have turned off their communication to everyone. Working with clients who offer little in the way of words in their session, can cause many clinicians to feel incompetent...as though they are not doing a good job helping the client speak up. Rather than blame yourself, talk to your client about it. Talk about how communication was handled in their home. Ask them if they decided to quit talking because no one was listening anyway. Explore their communication style and help them learn to express themselves.

DESIRE 2: To Be Affirmed

It feels nice to have people notice us, notice what we say and do. Unfortunately for many people in dysfunctional homes, they are noticed for their faults. As a therapist, the part of my job I love the best is affirming people. I love to point out how they've progressed in therapy, cheer them on when they try to make changes in their life, and affirm the pride they feel when they have made strides.

Being noticed for what we've done well by others is an important desire.

The Laasers highlight that "We long to have parents, friends, teachers, and mentors in our lives who also notice what we do well. People in our lives provide the feedback we need to develop our self-awareness about how we are doing in the world. Affirmation tells us that we are doing well and to keep it up." (Laaser, pg. 21) Those people who have not received affirmation end up doing two things; they learn to lie and they try to be perfect. When someone can't be themselves or they fear they will lose someone important if they are honest, that person will either try to be perfect so they feel loved and accepted, or they lie to please their loved one. This dynamic causes clients to lose their individual authenticity.

DESIRE 3: To Be Blessed

Feeling blessed is a warm, nurturing feeling people experience when someone tells them they are loved. To be blessed means "we don't have to do anything; we are loved for being just who we are. A blessing happens when someone lets you know that you are a very special person in their life. They love you, they are proud of you, and they want to be with you...When we are blessed, we don't have to do anything; we are loved for being just who we are." (Laaser, pg. 25)

People also feel blessed by God, knowing that He loves them just the way they are, not by what they do. Just existing is enough. Sadly, too many people have been criticized or ignored and never felt blessed by the people in their lives. These clients will come into our counseling office exhibiting loneliness, sadness, disconnection from others, and feeling a lack of self-worth. As compassionate, caring therapists, we can nurture this feeling of being blessed by offering unconditional positive regard.

What does unconditional positive regard look like in the counseling setting? I have many clients dealing with sexual abuse and some of them have lived very promiscuous lives, chosen abortions and have made choices they are ashamed of. It's important for me to be a "blank slate" for that client as they tell their story and as they allow me to dig deep into their shame. It's imperative to not judge, criticize, or shame the individual because of their mistakes. Having unconditional positive feelings toward the client means we feel genuine care for them and clients, then, feel the warmth we have to offer which allows a healthier sense of self-esteem to emerge.

Be aware of your body language which can also indicate to your clients how you are really feeling. Clients read our bodies all the time and we all know that if we sit with our arms crossed over our body, this posture can be interpreted as being bored, judging and "closed off." Be careful how you are communicating and consider treating your clients as a blessing.

DESIRE 4: To Be Safe

"We all desire to be safe--to be free of all fears and anxieties. We want to know that we are materially secure--that we have food, and a place to live, and enough money to support ourselves. And we want to know that we are emotionally secure, that those around us are reliable, that those people who say they love us can be counted on to act lovingly." (Laaser, pg. 28)

As children grow, and if they felt safety in their family home, they will grow up feeling confident and be willing to try new things or take more risks. Unfortunately, those clients from dysfunctional and abusive homes, or homes where emotions are not talked about, don't feel safe. They will be less likely to try new things and may become controlling in their behaviors toward others, have high anxiety, carry a load of shame, and if there has been abuse, will lack trust of others and themselves.

Judgment has no place in the counseling setting.

The abuse will also make adult relationships difficult and many will struggle with appropriate and healthy boundaries. When clients feel unsafe in their environment, they have learned to worry about everything...other people, money, relationships, work, and the list goes on. Safety is critical to healing. Offering a place of safety in our counseling office helps the individual learn to trust others and in turn to ultimately learn to trust themselves.

DESIRE 5: To Be Touched

Professional practitioners understand how important touch is for people. We know that babies cannot thrive without it. According to Laaser's book, "The desire for touch has two forms of expression. First we all have a desire to be sexually touched. That is a part of our human nature, and God put it there so that we will be fruitful and multiply. Second, we all have the desire to be touched in nonsexual ways. A problem arises when these two desires get confused. The desire for sexual touch is the energy inside of us to be productive, passionate, and creative...The sex drive is not evil, but it can be expressed in sinful ways when we don't follow God's design for healthy sexuality...The second form of the desire for touch is the desire for nonsexual touch. We all have a desire to be touched skin to skin, and this kind of touch doesn't have to lead to sex." (Laaser, pg. 33, 34)

However, in my practice, I have heard difficult stories from many men and women who lived in unhealthy homes where sexual touch was inappropriate and hurtful. Many children growing up in addictive homes have experienced inappropriate touch, boundary-less touch, whether physical or sexual. We know how difficult this can be as the children grow into adults and their understanding of healthy touch is warped. For some, they are fearful of any kind of touch; while others may crave enormous amounts, to the degree of sexual addiction and/or promiscuity.

As therapists, we struggle with whether or not to touch our clients. We have to be careful to determine when and if touch is appropriate. What I've learned is that it's important to help our clients realize what healthy touch looks like and ask for that from their own safe loved ones. Caution must be paramount when deciding if touch from a therapist is appropriate. Always ask the client first before touching and allow the client to say "No." I've found it best to not hug or touch a client unless they have initiated it. But be careful, many clients with codependency issues have unclear boundaries. For some, touch can have a sexual meaning to them when in fact that is not what you as a clinician intended it to mean. Encourage clients to get safe touch from safe people.

DESIRE 6: To Be Chosen

This need is universal in that we all need to feel chosen. We want to feel chosen by a mate, chosen to be a friend to someone, chosen to be included as part of a team, and chosen to be the next employee for a job. When you are not chosen, you create distorted beliefs about yourself that are not consistent with whom God has created you to be: I am not enough, I am not lovable, and I fall short of others. You desire to be chosen for who you are, and yet many of you go to great lengths to be things you are not in order to be chosen." (Laaser, pg. 36)

Clients often get confused and believe they will finally be chosen if they look or act a certain way. They may believe if they have the right body, the right clothes, the right material things like house and car, then they will be accepted and chosen by others. These are false and superficial ways to feel chosen. It's very sad that we strive for this desire and yet we get lost in our cultural ways and believe that looks and material things will make us more desirable. When codependents lose sight of who they are, they interact with others without authenticity, usually because they feel they need to become someone else to be desirable to others.

As therapists, helping clients identify what being chosen in a healthy way really means can be a challenge. Helping them realize that they are good enough just the way they are is a part of our task to help clients. It will be helpful to encourage clients to identify where and when they felt chosen. It may be difficult for them to identify, but continue to talk with them about people who have had a positive impact on their lives. When we help them identify a time and place where they felt chosen, this will help the individual build self-esteem and truly come to believe that they are enough regardless of how they look or what they do.

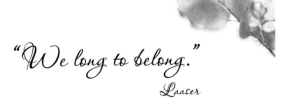

"We long to belong."

Laacer

DESIRE 7: To Be Included

Think back to a time when you were a young kid. We all had a need to be included within a certain group of friends, a church, our neighborhood, our home and family. But many people have experienced rejection and exclusion. This experience is very painful and yet common for many of our clients.

"The desire to be included is related to the desire to be chosen. This desire, however, is broader. We desire to be included in fellowship with God and with others. We long to belong. This desire is about community. We long to be a part of something larger than ourselves.

It helps us feel that we are not alone and gives us a sense of well-being. This sense of belonging gives us a feeling of needed security. Belonging has all kinds of emotional, physical and spiritual benefits." (Laaser, pg. 38)

Within an unhealthy family, too many people have felt as though they don't belong. They may feel they have taken on the role of the "black sheep," "misfit" or "scapegoat" and those roles do not feel inclusive. As therapists, it's important for us to help the client find ways and situations where they have been involved in their family or in their friendships. We may have to dig deep to find somewhere in their history where this was true. Inviting them to be a part of a codependency group you hold in your office can be helpful. Or encourage them to get involved in Al-Anon or another kind of support group. As their network of people grows through recovery, this need will eventually be met through many groups or connections with others.

IN SUMMARY: While living in dysfunctional families many clients may not have received any of these desires of the heart. Their needs were not met because the unhealthy person in their life demanded priority. The narcissism of unhealthy families leaves people yearning for connection. As you work with codependency, keep these desires in mind. Help the client focus on getting these needs met. Help them search for safe, healthy people who can love them and accept them. We can offer some help as therapists by being sensitive and loving toward our clients in every counseling setting and it can go a long way to providing hope and healing for those desires of the heart that were not met as children growing up.

Step 3: Safety, Support & Growth

- ## IDENTIFY SAFE PEOPLE

   Who are safe people and how do we know they are "safe?" This question is answered by Cloud and Townsend as they identify three criteria to consider when looking for safe people. They believe safe people will:

   ✓ Draw us closer to God
   ✓ Draw us closer to others
   ✓ Help us become the real person God created us to be

   Safe people, according to Cloud and Townsend, are those who live by their spiritual and Godly convictions and values. They have a template (The Ten Commandments) that direct their lives. Safe people encourage us, believe in us, and love us, as well as draw us closer to others by helping us to be more open and authentic. These people are truthful to us about our attitudes and behaviors and call us to be better individuals.

   God has created us to have a purpose. Safe people encourage that. Life is about learning what that purpose is and for many of us finding that purpose has been a long, arduous road. People we trust and who are safe are those that have OUR best interest in mind, not theirs. They value who we are and get excited for our progress and growth. They support us in whatever endeavors we strive for and trust us to make the right decision for ourselves.

Safe people have many positive qualities and I'm highlighting those attributes here:

✓ Keep your confidence - in other words, they are willing to keep your issues between the two of you and not gossip or share information with others, even if the codependent does not ask for confidentiality.

✓ Accepting and understanding - they are not judgmental and harsh about your situation. They are understanding and kind and accepting without shaming. Safe people understand how difficult decisions can be and they understand that everyone makes mistakes. They honor and value people even if they have made some poor choices. They do not ridicule, tease, criticize, or harass.

✓ Dependable and healthy - these are people with whom the codependent can rely on. They have balance in their life, they are emotionally stable, and their life is generally in order. We know we all have issues and there are times in our lives where things are chaotic, but overall they seem to have their act together.

✓ Honest and truthful - these people will be honest with the codependent in a kind and compassionate way. The safe person will help identify when the codependent is in denial or making excuses for their behavior. They are real and authentic with the codependent and tell them the truth with love.

Safe people have our best interest in mind.

✓ Healthy boundaries - friends who have healthy boundaries know when to say "No, I can't talk now," or "I feel uncomfortable with how much you're doing for someone." They understand what clear boundaries mean and how they look.

✓ Working on their own "issues" - They know how important continual growth is for everyone and they strive to learn new things, understand healthy relationships, and share their knowledge with us.

✓ Acknowledge our experiences - These safe people don't minimize our problems or try to fix us or fix the problems. They understand and can stay objective.

HOW CAN WE HELP? I spend time with my clients discussing and defining "safe" people. Establishing these connections are often very difficult because people with codependency issues may have isolated themselves from others. Isolation is a self-protective measure so the client doesn't need to explain themselves to others. They may have been challenged in the past by other people suggesting they may be doing too much for their family, kids, and/or spouse.

I will encourage them to reach out to people they believe they can trust. We will talk about those experiences of reaching out and how helpful it was for them. We will talk about the mistakes they may have made trusting someone who wasn't safe. Psycho-education and awareness work well in addressing the issues of safe people.

• **BUILD SUPPORT**
Because support groups have been so helpful for so many people, I encourage my clients to get into a group right from the start of counseling if they haven't already done so. I know many people are resistant to self-help groups, but the group setting offers so much support and basic self-care strategies. There are support groups for codependency such as Codependents Anonymous (CoDA), Al-anon/Alateen, Adult Children of Alcoholics (ACoA) and Celebrate Recovery, a Christian and Bible-based

group. All these groups are based on the Twelve-Step Program model of Alcoholics Anonymous (AA).

Those people who have attended groups before therapy already have a great start to their healing as the groups help individuals learn to focus on themselves, not others. These groups offer great strategies for living in relationships with other people who are unhealthy or addictive. Here, positive feedback is given, denial is broken, and learning to set boundaries and speaking the truth will be beneficial for the codependent. Slogans that many people find helpful include, "Live and let live," "One day at a time," "You didn't cause it, you can't control it, and you can't cure it." People attending these groups also learn that they are not alone in their struggles and there is help for them.

Be aware that many codependents will resist this idea. This can be an opportunity to talk to them about turning to others for help and allowing others to be a part of their lives. It addresses the isolation factor so many face. Learning to trust others and not have to "figure it out for themselves" brings relief. They didn't have a model from which to learn that there are safe, dependable people who can help them and some of these things are better taught through group interaction. Along with the counseling, the client is getting a lot of great information and support from both places (groups and therapy) to try out their new thoughts, feelings and behaviors.

Even if good support is available, many codependent people have learned to be totally independent and self-sufficient and have had trouble depending on others. Most of the people in their lives have been very undependable and untrustworthy. The trust level for these clients is very low and it's hard for them to trust that you could possibly care to help them. They may believe you have some ulterior motive that would serve your needs rather than their needs. So opening up and being real with a therapist is a difficult thing for them to do.

HOW CAN WE HELP? Encourage your client to start small...focus on only one person they can identify who is safe and they can trust. Ask them, "Who in your personal life, or at work, can you depend on and share your concerns with who will also keep your confidences?" Give them time to think and also time to try asking for help or sharing personal information with someone. I have found they will eventually come up with at least one person; they just need help identifying whom to choose. Throughout the counseling process, I will check in periodically to ask about building that support network to see that they have at least started the process. They will find much relief to not hold on to any more secrets alone and will learn that supportive people can help lift the burden they are carrying.

- **IDENTIFY & EXPRESS EMOTIONS**

People with codependency have learned to turn off their feelings and/or they are highly emotional. For those who are numb to feelings, I help them learn to identify new emotions. My hope is to help bring out the emotion and release them. Unfortunately many people with codependency have been so focused on others they don't know what or how to feel.

If the client grew up in an overly emotional home, they have learned to hold in their feelings or have not

JUST A FEW CODEPENDENT EMOTIONS

1. Anger/ Resentment
2. Powerlessness
3. Grief/Sadness & Disappointment
4. Anxiety
5. Hyper-Vigilance
6. Depression
7. Shame
8. Guilt
9. Hurt

learned how to express them in healthy ways. For example, if anger was explosive in their home, they may be reluctant to allow anger to come up because they don't want to be like that explosive family member. Others will have difficulty managing their feelings and they vomit their feelings all over anyone and everyone and abuse their loved ones.

When growing up in chaotic homes, much like those with any kind of addiction and abuse, the person with codependency is set up to be anxious, hyper-vigilant, and constantly on-guard. As children, their central nervous systems have been on high alert, ready to fire at any moment. The uncertainty and unpredictability of their situation keeps them highly focused on their surroundings, to the detriment of understanding their own wants and needs.

For those who had little help expressing emotion or saw no emotion expressed in their family system, they will have issues identifying feelings and don't have the vocabulary for them. Once we tap into their emotions, however, many feel enormous amounts of sadness and pain, anger, loneliness and resentment, etc. that they've carried with them for years and possibly decades.

HOW CAN WE HELP? In every session I'm thinking about emotions and want to help clients learn how to identify them. I will ask them to identify a feeling or two that they have experienced over the past week. For some clients I offer suggestions about what they may have been experiencing and ask them to choose one that fits best.

For those who are highly emotional and thrive on chaos, learning to manage those emotions will be important. First they need to understand their body and notice when feelings begin to churn. In our sessions, as those feelings come up, I will encourage them to focus on where in their body they feel the emotions. Then we discuss what to call that feeling. Codependents don't always have a vocabulary for affect, so we'll need to help them with this new language.

One technique I recommend is keeping a log of emotions throughout the day, learning to count to ten or take a break before expressing themselves. The key is to find a distracting strategy for your client so that they can manage their emotions and avoid sudden outbursts which can be destructive.

Following is a list of some of the most common emotions clients will bring into their sessions.

1. ANGER/RESENTMENT

We'll see the codependent either not exhibiting or expressing anger at all or expressing anger all over the place. For some people, they fear anger and they don't want to feel it because they are afraid they will get out of control much like others in their home growing up. Or they have few other emotions because anger becomes their "feeling of choice." In other words, they don't express other emotions because anger is their most prevalent one.

I've learned from personal experience as well as professionally that anger can be a secondary emotion. It may be the emotion that comes up first, but often underneath anger are other, more difficult to express emotions, such as fear, sadness, loneliness, and disappointment.

Let me give you an example. If someone jumps out at you from behind the door, you may get very angry. It's the first response. But this may be a defense mechanism for feeling something else. If the person takes some time to process it, they might realize that what they truly felt was fear. Anger was a default emotion.

So as practitioners, our job is to help them identify their emotions and learn to express them appropriately. Help the client express anger appropriately and without hurting others, but also help them to identify other feelings underneath that anger.

Resentment is something we all feel. However, many may be unaware of how resentful they actually do feel. These people have trouble saying "No" to others and rather than be direct and honest about how they feel, they become resentful which they keep inside. This then can become passive-aggressive behavior that shows up through sarcasm and bitterness.

Learning to identify and express emotions will improve emotional intimacy.

HOW CAN WE HELP? I suggest journaling to my clients and they can either journal daily or I also suggest to write for 20 minutes without picking up their pens. This allows the unconscious to come up in their journaling and they will find other stuffed feelings come to the surface. When they write without thinking, they are often surprised what comes up. I then have them read their letters in their next session to process what they had experienced.

Other options include talking to the "empty chair" in their session with you to release some of these difficult emotions. Notice their body language when you ask them to do this. Often you will observe them shrink into their chair out of fear or guilt. They may actually feel what it was like for them as a child to face someone with whom they couldn't talk to directly. Again, process this experience for them.

Another helpful intervention I suggest is to role-play ways in which they could express themselves. I will often play the role of the client and they take on the role of the "other person." I will offer ideas about how to express thoughts and emotions to someone. This has been very helpful for many of my clients and they will write down ideas to use later at home.

I take quite a bit of time in counseling to go over this emotional expression. Helping others express themselves for the first time and watching their transformation is very satisfying.

2. POWERLESSNESS

People struggling with codependency may have tried in vain to change other people and when change didn't happen, they felt powerless. This powerless feeling is what often brings clients into counseling. Their inability to control another person becomes exasperating and exhausting for them. So they seek outside help to gain the control they so desperately desire.

When growing up in difficult situations, children learn to control many facets of their environment as a way to alleviate anxiety. And part of their environment involves trying to control people. When kids take on the role of the adult and the adult is the child, children begin to believe they have power. They readily take on this extra responsibility.

However, as they become adults, others in their lives are not happy to have them try to control their lives and the codependent adult becomes overwhelmed and disillusioned. They become angry and resentful and feel a sense of powerlessness. Why are their old ways of controlling things not working, they wonder. Many people turn to counseling hoping to learn how to get others to do what they think is best only to realize they are the only one they can change.

The truth is we are powerless over much in life.

HOW CAN WE HELP? These issues give clinicians a great opportunity to educate and help clients understand the feeling of powerlessness. It's a chance to help them learn that the only person they ultimately have control over is themselves. Expect to encounter anger and frustration as clients learn these new concepts as they won't like to hear they can't control others. It's an important aspect of healing for codependency because once clients realize they can live life with powerlessness and allow others to direct their own lives, they will find relief. We all are powerless over many aspects of our lives and we can learn to be okay with that!

Talking about boundaries is important in the early stages of recovery from codependency. I use the Hoop Exercise (see page 155) to educate clients about who and what they have control over. And this concept will need to be reviewed throughout the process of recovery as different relationships are reviewed within counseling.

Helping the client redirect their focus from others to themselves can be a great challenge. However, as they do this and zero in on changing their own behavior, they will reclaim their power and realize what they have missed by being so focused on others.

3. GRIEF, SADNESS & DISAPPOINTMENT

In unhealthy relationships and throughout life, our clients, and all of us for that matter, have experienced an enormous amount of loss. For codependents, the loss of their relationships they thought were healthy is hard to face. I also hear how disappointed they are in themselves for allowing the dysfunction to go on for so long. Many feel the loss of a dream...a dream of a healthy marriage or healthy relationships. They feel a loss of self (or loss of their soul) as they've given up their dreams and lives for others. These losses are very important to process.

Codependency is a sad and lonely experience. However, as they process their pain and learn new strategies for living their lives in a way to please themselves rather than others, they will find new hope and excitement. As they process through these difficult emotions, the sadness and grief will lift. And as they build their self-esteem, their disappointment will transform into acceptance...acceptance of their unhealthy past, and acceptance of what is to come.

HOW CAN WE HELP? I encourage my clients to really feel their feelings. Let the sadness come up, along with the grief. I encourage them to cry and give themselves permission to release these feelings. Helping them through the grief cycle will be important. Just be there to help them through this pain, offering unconditional love and concern, which for many people may be the only real care and concern they've ever felt in their lives. It's a big responsibility as a therapist, but a very rewarding one as well.

4. **ANXIETY**

    As I mentioned earlier, many people living in dysfunctional homes have learned to be on high-alert. They are very sensitive to their surroundings and respond with hyper-vigilance. What this means is that physically their stomach may be churning, their muscles tight and painful, their mind whirling with all kinds of obsessive thoughts, along with feeling highly reactive emotions to experiences and people.

Learning to relax can improve mental health.

Those who have lived with dysfunction all their lives are very familiar with anxiety. They may believe everyone feels nervous all the time. It will be important for therapists to identify anxiety and help them learn to release and manage this emotion. Once they learn to relax and feel calm, they never want to go back to those uncomfortable and sometimes frightening feelings again.

HOW CAN WE HELP? I have found using an assessment scale is important to determine the level of anxiety that the client may be experiencing. We will then discuss ways in which to relieve this stress such as a visualization and meditation and muscle relaxation exercises. If medication is indicated, we will discuss this option as well. All of these therapies will be very helpful to relieve high anxiety.

I will always talk about to them about their nutrition. So many people eat or drink foods with high caffeine levels and when they have high levels, the body and central nervous system is on high alert, ready to fire at any moment, causing more tension and anxiety. So we'll talk about what they ingest into their body and learn to wean off those anxiety-producing foods and drinks.

I also suggest that the client try to sit still for a time to allow the body to learn to relax. I suggest they set the timer for a couple minutes to start. Then increase the time over the week, allowing their body to learn to be still. This can be a very difficult exercise for many people with codependency because their natural tendency (due to learned responses) has been to be on guard, active, moving continuously. Many clients are constantly busy...busy from morning until night. And staying busy is a great anxiety reliever. However, busyness gets in the way of intimacy with family and friends, and eventually becomes exhausting. Sitting still when the client is used to moving constantly can be a challenge, but it is also a great reward in the long run as they learn to relax and enjoy their quietness.

I have found visualizing a safe place, as I do for all EMDR sessions, can be helpful as well (see page 163). Encourage the client to close their eyes, visualize a place that is comforting and safe, taking it all in through their senses. I'll ask, "What do you see? What do you hear? What do you feel on your body? What do you smell?" Any way to let their senses be activated is important. I believe as we teach relaxation through understanding their body, their food, and through visualization, they can now have a different template from which to look at anxiety.

And as always, we know that exercise is a great stress and anxiety reliever. We will discuss options for them and encourage weekly exercise.

5. HYPER-VIGILANCE

Hyper-vigilance is a coping mechanism for many who have experienced abuse and unhealthy environmental issues. Because of their unsafe environments and unsafe people, codependents have learned to take a pulse on the people and situations around them. They become hyper-focused on their surroundings trying to decipher who is safe and who is not. They assess how others are acting, and whether or not their environment is out of harm's way. Sometimes their instincts are on target and sometimes they are not.

Hyper-vigilance causes exhaustion.

This intense awareness is exhausting and you will hear them complain about how tired they are. Client's who experience these feelings have a difficult time relaxing and enjoying themselves. And more importantly, many codependents can become seriously ill from the anxiety. I know some clients who have been diagnosed with cancer, heart problems, thyroid problems, fibromyalgia and other serious ailments, so don't take this hyper-vigilant quality lightly.

Hyper-vigilance may have been very effective in keeping them safe as a child if they were truly in danger, so in that regard it's been a great coping strategy. But it ultimately causes difficulty in relationships because they fear getting close to others. As clients realize what people and places are safe for them and begin to set boundaries along the way, they can learn to honor themselves and relax in the moment.

HOW CAN WE HELP? What I've encouraged my clients to do with this emotional reaction is to experiment with the next family event. For example, if the holidays are coming up and they expect they will be with family, I encourage them to take an emotional step back instead of reacting as they normally would. What that means is to notice what is going on around them, how people are interacting and responding to one another and just observe. Notice the roles each person takes on. And very importantly, notice what feelings are coming up for them. Taking a step back helps them to feel more in control of themselves and less a victim or reactionary in typical family interactions. It's very interesting for them to realize and then learn strategies to relax and become proactive in their family relationships.

When the client returns to their session the following week, we process what that family experience was like. We revisit the concept of safe people and help them identify who in their environment truly is safe for them. We'll talk about their experience and we brainstorm ideas for self-care.

6. **DEPRESSION**

It's helpful for clients to realize that depression is a normal emotion and we all feel depressed from time to time. However, when you have a client living in an unhealthy or toxic environment, it's important to assess for chronic depression and assess for suicidal ideation. Many codependent people have experienced lots of depression and have had little or no treatment for it. If medication is indicated, I will encourage them to talk with their doctor. However, if they have no suicidal ideation, I will suggest to them to try some of the therapy techniques first. They may find the interventions to be very helpful.

I also assess for dysthymia which is a chronic, low-grade type of depression that persists for more than two years. Many children growing up with abuse, alcoholism, or chronic mental health issues may have constantly felt down with little joy. Help clients understand dysthymia as well.

I've noticed, however, that often as clients address their codependency issues and learn to live in a healthier manner, their depression will lift. As they make changes and see positive results from the other interventions we've tried, they become excited about this new change, this new way of living. It's a great part of the therapy as you see your clients learn to live life with optimism and healthy interactions with their loved ones.

HOW CAN WE HELP? There are several psychological scales you will find helpful to assess for depression. I will have the client take an assessment at the beginning of our therapy process and then go back over it several sessions later to see what improvements they have made. Also, Cognitive Behavioral Therapy approaches are helpful whether it's tracking the depressive feelings and capturing negative thoughts.

I have also found that EMDR is very helpful to address the negative self-take and negative beliefs. Not only does it address the targeted situations that were harmful to the client, but also addresses the negative beliefs that have developed out of the dysfunction that the client has lived.

7. SHAME

Shame, for many, literally stops them in their tracks because they are so ashamed of themselves, ashamed of a mistake they've made, a decision that didn't turn out well, words they've spoken and behaviors they've exhibited. Shame can cause clients to feel stuck and they will have difficulty making progress in their therapy. If this happens, it's wise to address it and deal head on with the shame that debilitates them.

Abuse and neglect contribute to shameful feelings. Children learn they are not important to their family and have experiences which include being called worthless, bad, a whore, to blame, unloved, unwanted and many other horrible things. This kind of emotional and verbal abuse just destroys the self-esteem of these kids and as they grow into adults they continue to carry this shame with them.

You may hear from clients, "I felt so stupid after I left that party. Why did I say those things or why did I do that?" They revisit every move they have made and every word they've spoken. In their relationships they may feel unworthy of friendships, love, compassion and concern, no matter how hard another person tries to encourage them.

HOW CAN WE HELP? Notice the client's body language. Often you'll see a client, when experiencing shame, slump their shoulders, drop their head down, and even "zone out." Take time to stop and acknowledge the shame. Ask about where they feel the shame in their bodies. Ask about the negative self-talk going on in their head, for example, "I'm a bad person," "I'm worthless," and "I'm to blame."
Like all emotions, identifying shame is the first step. As they learn more about shame, they are often surprised that they have lived their entire life with it and it's a stubborn feeling to repair.

Here is where I use a lot of positive reinforcement. I highlight those things they are doing well, even if they resist (and they will). I encourage clients to read up on shame, understand the emotion and start treating themselves as valuable.

Next I will address that little kid inside them. I ask that they imagine themselves as a little child, elementary school aged or younger, and I inquire what they didn't get from the adults in their life. Or in the case of abuse, what they should <u>not</u> have gotten from them. Then I have them ask that child what they would have needed then. We take time to visualize what they desired. If there were words they needed to hear, I will say those words aloud. Hearing the words from someone outside of themselves often brings them to tears. I ask them to take those words in and start to believe them. This will take many sessions to do because the shameful messages are so engrained in their being.

I encourage them to use this strategy outside of the counseling setting as a way to counteract shame. I suggest that they talk to their inner child and treat him or her with love and kindness. Then, I ask them to imagine their inner child taking in all the positive statements and words and visualize how they may feel hearing them.

Another simple step for alleviating shame that I recommend to my clients is reading affirmation books. I believe these positive messages can counteract the negative ones they may have grown up hearing and believing and begin to reprogram their self-talk.

If your client is a Christian, it is helpful to remind them that God doesn't make mistakes. We know the scriptures tell us that they were known well before they were born and that they have an important job to do here on earth. For some, this reminder is very helpful. It may take some time, but my hope is that by repeating this message, eventually they will come to believe that they do in fact matter.

8. GUILT

Guilt can be a positive emotion because it keeps us doing the "right" thing, staying on the correct path and reminding us not to go against our morals and values. However, for some people guilt has been a burden to bear throughout their lives.

You will find guilt come up for many codependent people when they are trying to make changes. If they are trying to set new, healthy boundaries, they feel guilty. If they talk to someone in a new way, they feel guilty. If they don't care-take someone, they will feel guilty. Remind clients that whenever they make a change, they will feel guilt. That's fine. Just keep going forward in spite of the guilt.

Healthy guilt keeps us on the right track.

For some people, their lives have been full of "shoulds." "I should have done this" or "I should have said that." When they have lived their lives with "should's" they become very guilt-ridden. Often these expectations come from other people in their lives as well as from their religious upbringings. If a client has had a more legalistic church life, they may struggle with the guilt of the church's teachings. In their families, it's possible the rules were inflexible and rigid.

HOW CAN WE HELP? Awareness is key before change can be made. Help the client challenge their guilty feelings. Help them determine if that is a belief they want to adhere to or let go.

As a way to alleviate guilt, I encourage my clients to have a safe friend to call when their guilt gets the best of them. They need another person to encourage them as they make these changes because their overwhelming feelings could sabotage their success and their desire to try the new behaviors. The support they receive from these people can help battle this stubborn emotion.

9. HURT

Due to the narcissism of the addict, the codependent person experiences hurt and pain because their needs and desires have been neglected or abused. Both extremes cause an enormous amount of pain. As I've worked with clients, I notice that hurt is usually not the presenting emotion. The presenting emotion usually is sadness and/or anger as the codependent hasn't gotten to the deep pain their unhealthy upbringing has caused. Many of our clients will have stuffed those feelings or avoided them all together. Many clients have denied their hurt because it's too difficult for a child, and even an adult, to believe their loved ones have caused so much distress. I believe it's a coping strategy as a way to survive the deep-seeded suffering.

For others, often, hurt is covered up with anger. Some people remain stuck in their anger and it may take time for them to address the hurt underneath. This, too, is another way in which to cope.

HOW CAN WE HELP? As clients address the feelings of hurt, they begin to "thaw out." This means that once they realize they have these deep hurts and allow themselves to experience the emotions, their pain will rise up. As practitioners, we know these feelings are painful and rarely do any of us like to feel these feelings. But being there for the client as they become acquainted with the pain is important. We will need to be there to witness their pain, hold their pain, and help them move through their pain.

Encourage clients to feel the feelings and help them to talk about that experience. For this type of emotion, I will use the "little child" again, encouraging the client to picture themselves as that young child back there in that painful experience. (I'll have them bring in a picture of themselves at that age to remind them how little they were.) This seems to help enormously when they see themselves at that young, vulnerable age.

We talk about what they missed. If they could have had it just the way they needed it, I have them envision what that would look like. Maybe it was a hug, an arm around their shoulders, an understanding adult who could have listened to them. Again, EMDR is very helpful for working through these emotions and the negative cognitions that accompany them.

EMOTIONS IN SUMMARY: I use the Life Development Project (see page 144) to begin addressing emotions. As the client tells me their story, I frequently ask how they had felt around certain situations. If you hear expressions like, "I don't know," or "It didn't really bother me," or "I was fine," usually this can indicate that the client has little connection to their emotions. Encourage them to be honest and create a safe setting for them. You may have to give the client ideas to get started. For example, you might advise them "If that happened to me, I certainly would feel hurt," or "What do you think your friend would feel if that happened to them?"

I encourage my clients from the intake session on forward to be honest with me about what they are feeling. If they are unhappy with counseling or don't agree with something I've said, I ask them to express that. I want them to know that my office is a safe place to practice expressing any emotion. And don't let their negative feelings get under your skin so you become defensive. You may have a different perspective and not agree with them, but don't argue. Allow the client an opportunity to express themselves honestly and compliment them as they try their new skills with you...the safe person in their life.

When safe people have been identified, I encourage the client to practice their new skills of communicating feelings. I help them understand that their presentation matters. Timing, too, is important. So we prepare for an interaction with someone so they can practice their new skill.

I encourage them to set up a time to talk with the person. We discuss other healthy tactics in presenting their feelings, which includes awareness of their volume and tone of voice. I tell them that an aggressive approach will only put the other person on the defensive and soft spoken words are easier to hear...keep contempt and other negative emotions under control. I encourage my client to be as open-minded as they can so they hear the other person's perspective. They don't have to agree. It's just an opportunity to get their emotions expressed. And one more important aspect of expressing themselves, I coach clients how to talk about the issue without blaming the other person using "I" statements and expressing emotions rather than criticism.

Here is an example of a conversation: "I would love to have a chance to talk with you sometime, soon. Can we get together for a conversation around 3:00 pm today?" Once the conversation has begun, the client could say, "I have been hurt and disappointed that we haven't had a date for a long time. I miss you. I would like to get something scheduled and I would love to have you organize it." There is no criticism of what they haven't done, just a request with love and compassion of what they'd like to have happen in the future. It takes practice and also courage. Trying new strategies will cause most people anxiety, but I encourage all my clients to keep going even though they are nervous.

My hope is that as clients understand their emotions and learn to express them appropriately, they will find healthy connections and deeper emotional intimacy with others.

- ## TEACH SELF-CARE

    We know that many codependents struggle with taking care of themselves due to feelings of guilt or selfishness, because they have learned to focus their attention on caring for others. I believe this strategy of self-care is critical to codependency recovery and it will be a challenge for clients to learn to do this for themselves.

    I spend many sessions talking with clients about their beliefs around self-care. For many people who grew up in unhealthy families, self-care was not modeled for them and in fact, many were told that their needs didn't matter. What they learned was that taking care of others was to be a priority because many of the adults in their lives were unable or unwilling to care for them. When a parent is unable, due to addictions or mental illness, the children learn to take on that role and not only care for the adults, but take on the responsibility of caring for their siblings. Their soul has been lost in this process.

    I also believe our culture contributes to this problem and women have generally been taught to care for others at their own expense. As wives and mothers, women give and give until they are completely depleted. I also see this in the church community because Christians are taught it is better to give than to receive. And typically the same people in the church are the ones who give and volunteer regardless of what they have going on in their personal lives. Sometimes this is a coping strategy to not face their personal issues, but often it's because no one modeled that caring for themselves was important.

Self-care is not selfish,

it's imperative!

As teachers and coaches, we can help our clients make themselves a priority. I accomplish this by assigning to my clients homework to start the self-care process which may consist of: resting for ten minutes per day, going to bed early if they're tired, saying, "No" to the demands of others, taking a bubble bath, or have a night out with a friend. Clients love this homework. They come back into their session so thrilled and proud of themselves that they've taken this positive step.

Balance is important in self-care and I remind my clients that they don't have to completely abandon caring for others, but to simply find the balance between the two.

HOW CAN WE HELP? I'm reminded of the analogy when you're on a plane and they advise you to put the oxygen mask on yourself first, before those you're caring for. This is true in life as well. One diagram I use to help clients understand the concept of balancing self-care is using the bucket example. I explain that all our buckets have holes in the bottom and there are many things that drain us of our resources and energy. For too many of us, however, our buckets are drained completely. The bucket is dry. The hole is enormous. You'll often see clients coming in to counseling at this drained stage of their lives. They are exhausted and don't have another ounce to give to anyone.

So we talk about what fills their bucket. How do they fill it? What energizes them? What do they love to do? What excites them and feels good? We brainstorm ideas and I encourage them to start filling their bucket in small ways, small actions that can start the process. I love talking, too, about reconnecting with God. Often if they begin praying, going back to church, starting a Bible study, they will begin to get filled up. Maybe they've given up a hobby, for example. Take back that hobby! It's a great reminder not only for our clients, but for ourselves. How empty is your bucket?

THE BUCKET

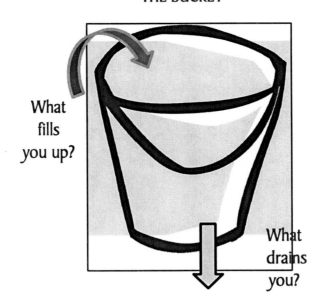

What fills you up?

What drains you?

- ## DETACH WITH LOVE

Detachment is a very difficult task for codependent people to do. They feel as if they are abandoning their loved one if they "let go." But healthy detachment is crucial to establishing healthy connections.

Our clients can still love the other person while allowing them the freedom to decide for themselves how to live their lives, though it's risky. When they let go, the loved one may be upset by the changes in the relationship. Anytime there is change, it causes upheaval. At the extreme, the loved one may decide to leave or abandon the relationship and we know this is a risk. Working through this issue of detaching and helping the client express their feelings with their loved one with love and respect, can smooth this detachment process out, hopefully with no one abandoning the relationship. Although this can be very difficult for those who have been abandoned many times in their lives, in the long run the health of the relationship will develop and all individuals involved can take responsibility for themselves and feel good about who they are and be free of oppressing one another.

Healthy Detachment looks like this:
- ✓ Releasing, or detaching from a person or problem with "love," not with spite or anger.
- ✓ Mentally and emotionally, and sometimes physically, disengaging themselves from unhealthy (and frequently painful) entanglements with another person's life and responsibilities and from problems they can't solve.
- ✓ Each person is responsible for him/herself knowing they can't solve problems that aren't theirs to solve and know worrying doesn't help.
- ✓ Involves living in the present moment, in the here and now, not the past or the future.

✓ Involves accepting reality – the facts. Admits when there are problems instead of ignoring those issues and denying them.

✓ Requires faith – in self, in God, and other people.

The rewards of detachment bring serenity and a deep sense of peace. It's possible to learn to give and receive love in self-enhancing, energizing ways and it can bring freedom to many peoples' lives. Finding freedom to live life without excessive feelings of guilt about or responsibility for others is a major accomplishment.

As I just mentioned, codependent people may fear being abandoned. And if they fear abandonment, they fear that setting boundaries, not coming to the rescue of their loved one, and letting go of others while also taking care of themselves will cause the loved one to leave. These fears are real. However, these relationships are strongly attached in unhealthy ways.

I do let my clients know that letting go and not taking care of their loved one in unhealthy ways is a risk. They could ultimately lose that person from their life, so they will have to choose whether or not to take that risk. In our sessions, however, we talk about and plan accordingly so as to lower the risk of that loss.

Because so many people struggle with "black and white" thinking, when they hear detachment, they think of leaving the person all together. Therefore, we have to remember to help them understand the "gray" areas. Detachment means not jumping in to help a loved one who can help themselves. We can emotionally encourage and support the other person, but we don't have to do for them what they can do for themselves. This is detaching with love.

In my experience, attachment with my mother was very unhealthy. I felt very independent and yet was emotionally attached. I felt what my mother felt. In fact, I had more feelings about my mother's life than I believe she did. When she was admitted for alcohol treatment in the late 1970s, I was so distraught and felt as though I was abandoning her. My true, authentic self didn't exist. Other peoples' feelings were my feelings. It was very sad and very painful.

Detaching with love brings relief to the codependent.

I tried to detach from my mother, and I ended up detaching completely. I didn't speak to her for one year. She was not invited to family birthdays and celebrations and I know it was terribly painful for her. I didn't know how to detach with love and ultimately the whole family was affected by my decision. My children did not have their grandmother with them to celebrate their events and I came to realize that I had made some painful decisions for many people. What I should have done was talk with her, explain to her I needed some time and space to understand and connect with myself. I didn't need to exclude her completely from family gatherings. It was a very sad time for us both, but it felt at the time my only option.

After a year, however, when I felt strong and self-confident, I wrote my mother a letter and we were able to mend our relationship. The greatest thing that came out of all that pain was a relationship with my mother that was mature. I was not relating to her as her child anymore. I was the confident adult I was meant to be and our relationship was on equal footing.

HOW CAN WE HELP? Together, with your client, determine what healthy detachment would look like for them. I have found that psycho-education is very helpful. I teach communication skills, and encourage them to speak up, speak to their loved ones directly and with honesty. We role-play to help them gain experience by expressing their thoughts and emotions using "I" statements.

Talk with your client about timing a discussion with a loved one and presenting your concerns with sensitivity. I suggest using the AA and Al-anon way of deciding when and if a conversation could happen. It's called the HALT Method, and if anyone is experiencing any of these, do not get involved in a deep or important conversation.

I also offer to have those tough conversations with loved ones in my counseling office, and provide whatever support and encourage-ment I can to help navigate through these relationship difficulties. Often learning new strategies can bring relief for all the people involved. Defining detachment with the client and discussing options will be a great

HALT METHOD
H ungry
A ngry
L onely
T ired

start. But again, know that this can be a tough step to make, so being open as a therapist to the client's timing will be important.

- **TEACH ASSERTIVENESS SKILLS**

Helping clients learn to assert themselves in effective, respectful ways will weave throughout the counseling process. For many codependents, their ability to ask for what they need and use assertiveness skills can be a real problem or even non-existent.

For people with low self-esteem, being assertive is a foreign concept. Unhealthy families have not shown the children how to do this appropriately and if they've tried, they may have been abused, ridiculed or abandoned.

Clients fall into the extreme ends of the spectrum, whether they are shy, timid or reluctant to ask for what they want and need and then there are others on the opposite end of the spectrum who can be demanding and controlling. Both extremes are problematic in relationships.

HOW CAN WE HELP? As we work through the issues of codependency, I'm always listening for areas of their life in which they've had successes, such as standing up for themselves in any situation. I want to acknowledge those abilities and encourage more assertiveness. Clients often have selective memory and don't realize that they've been assertive and asked for their needs. We just need to remind them!

If they have been demanding and controlling in their relationships, we discuss options to ask for their needs respectfully and with a caring spirit. Psycho-education can be helpful for these clients as well as looking at their history to understand how their controlling nature developed. Determining healthy coping strategies, rather than bossing others around, can often get their needs met better and be a relief for their family who has endured their abusiveness.

I have found role-play a very helpful strategy for the client to learn healthy assertiveness skills. I ask them to play the role of the "other person," and

I play their role. By focusing on a situation and learning the new words to use to assert themselves works well. I have had many people write down our ideas, even word for word, to help them practice when they get home.

Setting boundaries requires assertiveness skills, so we define together what boundaries they want to set and how best to present them. Talk to the client about their attitude and tone as they begin to present their viewpoint. Ask them to notice if they become defensive or edgy, or if they are irate or calm. Self-awareness is very important when defining how to present something new to another person.

Timing is important to consider when talking about difficult topics and I explain to clients to make sure they plan a time to discuss things when both parties are in a good place emotionally; for example, using the HALT method. Also, choose a time when the children are busy or away from the home. Children can cause too much distraction and frustration for both parties if the adults are interrupted. If the discussion gets too heated, the kids need to be out of the fray.

Determining a good place in which to have these conversations is important as well. For some clients, a particular room in their home that is neutral is a great place to start. Never argue or discuss issues in the bedroom as it may make the space seem "unsafe" to either person. I may also encourage clients to go to a public place so both people will keep themselves and their emotions under control.

Help the client strategize when, where, and how to ask for what they need and encourage them to assert themselves with a subject that in the past may have been intimidating. Some clients have had little experience with asserting themselves, so like many other areas of their recovery, the client may need clear, concise, healthy direction. This can be a very rewarding part of their counseling for both of you. It's wonderful to see your client take back their power and feel good about new tactics they have tried that get the results they are hoping for.

Step 4: Codependency Treatment Difficulties

Recovery from codependency has some particular reactions that you can expect to run across during therapy and it's important to be aware of these common traits. As clients are learning new skills and "trying on" new behaviors, they will usually go through a period of feeling incompetent. They may find their relationships are in more disarray initially and be concerned that these changes are only making matters worse, rather than better. Be sure to reassure them that whenever change happens, things may be more unsettled for a time. It's a normal part of the process and things will get better...it may just take some time and patience.

For example, if a client is trying to set boundaries with someone for the first few times, they will most likely struggle with how to address the issue, how to communicate their desire, and will probably feel very guilty in the process. Help them understand that like trying to learn something new, they will make mistakes and be unsure of themselves at first. Encourage them to keep trying and continue this new behavior even though they feel guilty. "Working through the guilt" will be an important step for them to take.

As these changes happen, family members may be angry and confused because they won't like the shift in the relationship. That, too, is normal. Help them see that these changes need to continue even though it feels difficult.

In terms of the emotional roller coaster they may experience, it could seem as though their feelings are extreme or out of control. It may be one of the first times they've expressed anger, for example, and as they tried to express the emotion, they were overly aggressive. I explain to my clients that they may go from one extreme to the other at first before they find a comfortable, balanced behavior or thought. Someone who was normally passive in their relationships and decides to assert themselves could seem "bossy" in their own eyes (as well as their family's eyes) as this new behavior feels so unnatural. Help your clients understand this dynamic to alleviate the guilt and shame they may feel if they've either hurt someone or been unsuccessful while trying a new approach to their relationships.

Hyper-focusing on others

is a common issue.

Often I see people come in to my office not understanding themselves or knowing who they are. They will complain about feeling lost or having no direction for their life. They may feel depressed or anxious and not sure why. They don't realize they have lived their life inauthentically or incongruently and have lived like that for so long, based on what they thought others wanted of them, they don't realize who they are. As Beattie suggests, the reality in terms of the individual's body, their thinking, feeling and behavior, is non-existent. Many have identified their own reality to what they want it to be which is false and fake as they may be living in a fantasy world. Often you, as their therapist, may experience confusion when talking with them because what they experience and what they tell you may look very different because their perceptions are so inaccurate.

If clients have a misconception of how they look, they can take on dysfunctional eating habits and become obese or anorexic. Perhaps their body language indicates that they're angry, but they insist they aren't. They are just so unaware because they've lost touch with their emotions and body.

Here are some other common obstacles you will face while dealing with codependency. I want to remind you that you will need to be patient. These hurdles can be dealt with and you can work through them with the client. Simply be aware and tuned in as you face these defense mechanisms:

- **RESISTANCE**

  We have all learned that resistance can be a common struggle when working with clients with many different issues. As we suggest different ways for the client to respond to other people in their life we may hear, "Oh, I can't do that. I'd feel too guilty." Or the client may not do their homework, and after we've explored that further, the client is feeling resistant to the new strategies. It's common to face resistance, but the best way to get around it is to go right through it.

  When working with a codependent person and because they can be struggling with denial, you will feel the resistance until the walls of denial come down. So take your time, pace with the client, and use psycho-education to help inform them about the addiction or the dysfunction in the family system (at this time, talk about the hoops, the three chairs, dysfunctional family systems, etc., coming up in future chapters). You may also want to recommend that they read codependent books to help them identify characteristics of the dysfunction.

  As trust builds and the client begins to feel more comfortable with you, talk about change and address any resistance that comes up. You may sense a hesitation from the client to go into a certain issue. Pay special attention to their fears around change.

When I'm working with a client who I sense is feeling resistant, I will often ask them to be aware of the feeling they are experiencing at that moment. Using the word "resistant" can trigger clients into shame to emotionally shut down. Another word I've suggested for clients might be "hesitation." I inquire about that hesitation and talk about how that has been a way to protect themselves from harm in their past which played a significant role in keeping them safe.

Pushing the client can have negative effects.

Walk alongside clients and be there for them as issues surface. I believe the clients have the answers within themselves and part of my therapy is helping them listen to their quiet voices within. As they begin addressing these intuitive ideas, they are tuning into themselves, which is a step in the healing direction toward self-trust.

- **NOT KNOWING WHAT THEY WANT OR NEED**

Because so many clients have focused their attention on others, rather than themselves, they may have difficulty knowing what wants or needs they have. A common response from my clients when asked what needs they have is, "I don't know." They seem genuinely surprised at the question. I have heard from clients that few people have ever inquired about what their interests or desires were. Many female clients have reported that they felt selfish when they think or do for themselves and it's uncomfortable. Here is where you can encourage and educate, as their needs do matter.

When I've worked with clients around their needs, I have them envision themselves as a little child. As I've discussed before, we talk about what they needed and help them envision that child getting his/her needs met. This visualization usually brings on emotions for the client as they think about nurturing that little child. It helps them get in touch with that vulnerability and I encourage them to listen to that child-like part of themselves.

Another approach I use involves taking charge of their time and their body. For many codependent people, they work hard, they accomplish much, and they feel exhausted. Their anxiety is high and they feel as though they have to move and must not sit still. I would encourage you to use the Relaxation Exercise (page 162) along with the Safe Place Exercise (page 163) to get started.

In order to learn to focus, one has to start small and practice. Initially sitting still for five minutes is asking a lot for some people. The client may notice how distracted they are, how fidgety their body is, how much anxiety and guilt they feel just focusing on themselves. I remain supportive no matter how long they can sustain this and ask that they try to sit for longer periods, working towards 30 minutes of stillness.

As you work with clients to help them understand themselves better, their wants and needs will become clearer. Baby steps.....

- **MINIMIZING**

As clients begin to address their issues, behaviors, thoughts and feelings, you may come up against minimization. For example, when they are asked how they felt about something and they've not had much practice with identifying emotions, you might hear, "It didn't bother me." Or they may say something like, "I didn't really care" or "It was no big deal." When faced with these obstacles, it will be important to carefully and respectfully check in with the client to be sure that is actually the case. These responses indicate the resistant nature the client is in. It's such a habit and a quick response that most codependents struggling with minimization will have to be reminded that those things maybe did matter and that what they felt was tough to experience and their situation was very painful.

Another example of minimizing, clients with codependency have trouble taking compliments. In the midst of my difficult codependent years, whenever I received a compliment my thoughts went directly to, "If they only knew..." It's very difficult for them to take these positive remarks. Don't give up, however. Help them realize their automatic responses and help them understand that this is a normal stage of codependency and it can change.

When you come up against minimization, address it by suggesting some other way to look at things or help them acknowledge what really did happen. You can do this by acknowledging to your client what your own feelings would probably be if you experienced something similar - giving them permission to feel those emotions as others might. Just keep in mind that this has been an important coping strategy that your client believes has worked well, so you will hear these minimizing statements through the counseling process.

As you work through the issues and address the codependency, minimization will diminish. It's part of the healing process and yet is an important one that needs attention.

- **DEFENSIVENESS**

   Many people have walls that can be hard to penetrate and the client may have difficulty letting down those walls. Those defenses have kept them safe for a long time and letting go of them can be terrifying. Be prepared for defensive reactions to questions you may ask the client and potential resistance to learning new ways of interacting with others. Or as you are trying to redirect the client to focus on their own issues, you may feel resistance here as well.

   Defensiveness has been a great strategy for codependents to keep others at a distance. This feels more comfortable for them as emotional intimacy feels awkward. You will run into this coping strategy often and it will be important to address this with them. Don't take their defensiveness personally, but be sure and identify the issue and help them learn to let people get closer to them.

   I have found that talking about this protective response using psycho-education can be very helpful and I will often teach The Three Chairs Exercise (see the next page). We discuss in more detail the "defensive" or "survivor chair" and how that stance was a self-protective practice to keep from being hurt. Understanding this can alleviate the shame many clients commonly experience and also help them be aware of and sympathetic of other's behavior.

   This exercise has been adapted from the Faithful and True women's intensive workshops and was originally developed by Marilyn Murray.

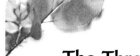

The Three Chairs Exercise

As the title suggests, three chairs are used: A child-sized chair, called the "Child" chair; a mid-sized chair which is hard and uncomfortable, called the "Survivor" or "Defensive" chair; and an oversized, beautiful, luxurious chair, called the "Wise" chair. As I discuss the different perceptions and beliefs we all experience at each stage, I ask the client to sit in the chairs, moving from one to another. Often we talk about a situation that they are struggling with and focus on that issue as they move back and forth.

- **CHILD CHAIR:** In the "Child" chair I ask them to think about how precious and blameless they were at this childish stage and how perfectly and wonderfully made they were. At this stage of life they are creating beliefs about themselves and their world based on their experiences.

Also at this stage, they haven't had much in the way of pain, with some exceptions of course. Here they are wide-eyed and eager to conquer the world. Many children have had their needs met; however, other children have had much difficulty.

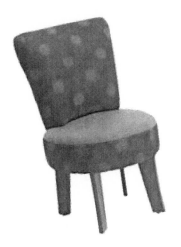

As the years pass, those positive and negative beliefs become powerful as they become the way in which they view the world. For example, if a parent was unavailable to meet their needs (i.e., a baby was left in its crib without food or diaper changing), they may learn through that experience that they "don't matter" or feel they are "a burden." If they've had positive experiences, they learned that they are capable and competent. What happens in those early years can impact them throughout their entire lives.

Explore with the client how they felt at this stage and how they imagine they would have felt if they can put themselves "back there" in their mind. Ask them to notice their thoughts, notice their feelings, and notice their body. What is all of that trying to tell them?

As life happens and hurt has been experienced, children learn to "put on their armor" and build a wall to protect themselves from further hurt. Now we move into the middle chair.

- **SURVIVOR/DEFENSIVE CHAIR:** As children grow older and experience pain, they learn to protect themselves and focus their attention to survive with as little pain as possible. The second chair is uncomfortable and hard and represents the resistance and defensiveness built up from pain and disappointment they have experienced as children. This is called the "Survivor" or "Defensive" chair.

Often addictions and codependency become the coping strategies many clients use to protect themselves and not feel the despair. They create messages and lies about themselves and others from their personal experiences. This position isolates them from others and they come to believe it's a protective place for them to be. At this point, I will point out that we all experience these feelings and yet some of our defenses look different.

In the defensive/survivor place the clients may act as though they don't care, regardless of what others have said to them. They are angry and frustrated much of the time and may use chemicals and other negative coping strategies as a way to keep people away from them to protect themselves. For codependents, they can live much of their lives here, as well as in their little "Child" chair which keeps the relationships they have very immature. They will waver back and forth between the chairs from time to time.

Again, have the client sit in the chair and feel the hardness of it. It will take them to a specific incident in their mind and make them aware of the defensive nature they put on to keep hurt away.

I then ask them to move to the next chair, which is the "Wise" chair. Have them sit in it and ask what they notice. What do they feel? What comes to mind? The experience of actually sitting in the chairs gives you great work to process. Let them talk about times in their lives where they have been in those "chairs."

- **WISE CHAIR:** The third chair is big and comfy and is called the "Wise" chair because people who are confident in themselves make decisions without guilt and shame. They are not defensive and when they have disagreements with others, they don't fall into self-blame. They can hear others' thoughts and feelings without feeling responsible for them and they know they are not responsible to fix things. They can be silly, laugh and feel peace and contentment. In this chair, they give themselves permission to feel their feelings without regret or shame.

In the "Wise" chair clients make good decisions because they can slow down the process for themselves and determine what the right decision is for them. They love themselves and can love others without getting triggered into unhealthy and overwhelming feelings. They know they do not have to take care of others in this chair unless they choose to do that and they don't feel guilt and a sense of responsibility for others. Their behaviors are chosen and not reactive, but rather proactive.

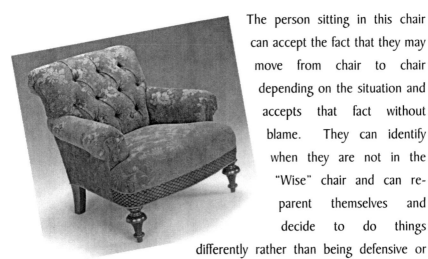

The person sitting in this chair can accept the fact that they may move from chair to chair depending on the situation and accepts that fact without blame. They can identify when they are not in the "Wise" chair and can re-parent themselves and decide to do things differently rather than being defensive or child-like. In this position, the individual can claim what is true for them, regardless how others feel.

Take time to go over their thoughts and feelings of being in each chair. This is a great way to help the client understand themselves and it reduces shame for many people because they realize that we all "sit" in all three chairs. It's helpful to work with the client to identify the pain they felt early on that prompted them to move to the "Survivor" or "Defensive" chair. As they learn what it takes to sit in the "Wise" chair, they now have a new template of what it can look like to live life authentically.

The visual of the chairs allows your clients to be more aware of their reactions to others, and they can imagine themselves in the "Wise" chair in the here and now. They can identify when they are feeling self-protective because they visualize the "Defensive" chair. They can identify when another person may be acting out of the "Defensive" chair and learn to respond accordingly and in a healthy way. My clients love this technique and grasp the concept very quickly and easily.

• TYPICAL REACTIONS TO LIFE CHANGES

Look for patterns that I've identified on the following pages. As you see them, be honest with the client but also take care in presenting them. Shame can be easily triggered in people struggling with codependency. A way I've gotten around that is to simply ask the client the question, "What patterns do you see?" Let them identify what they see and if you have other concerns, it can be brought up at that time. Don't tiptoe around issues, just be compassionate and cognizant of shame and understand how quickly that can be triggered for some codependents.

✓ **CLIENT'S FEAR:** Fear is something that can get in the way of their recovery. Because codependency has such a large component of fear, you will find codependents very apprehensive of change. Change can be seen to them as a threat, so remember that you may have to encourage, challenge, and nudge the client forward. Many clients have such anxiety and depression because the life they've lived has been hurtful, scary, and chaotic that their fear keeps them stuck.

For those codependents who have not said "No" to others, setting that boundary can also be terrifying for them. They may fear rejection from their loved one, or they have seen abandonment in other relationships, so their fear may be real. Sorting this out with them will help. For others, they may have legitimate fears of being physically or emotionally hurt. Asses for safety as you go along and you may have to define smaller steps for those clients with legitimate safety issues.

✓ **CLIENTS STAY STUCK:** For some clients, their unhealthy coping strategies have worked in the past, so they fall back to those strategies because it's familiar to them. It will take some time for the client to understand the new concept of focusing on themselves. And the anxiety of trying new ways of life can keep them stuck in their feelings. Don't stop! Keep going. If you as their therapist feel stuck, you can bet that the client is feeling the same way. Talk about it and make a plan to try something new to move forward.

Patience is challenging when clients are stuck!

✓ **CLIENT'S GUILT:** Most codependents (and others as well) are fearful they will hurt their loved ones if they try new approaches to their relationships. Be sure and let them know that whenever they change things up they will feel guilty. Help them first by becoming aware of the feeling, acknowledging that the guilt is there, but encourage them to keep moving forward in their recovery in spite of it. Working through guilt is important for all clients because we know as practitioners we will feel these feelings when we do something different in life.

✓ **CLIENT'S VERBAL REPETITION:** It's common to spend many sessions simply listening. Often people with codependency need to be heard and they are eager to share their stories. If you notice stories that seem scattered and repetitive, stick with the client as they will get to their point. Don't rush the process. To build trust, many clients need to be in charge of the counseling session for a time. I have noticed that as clients' lives become less scattered and they have learned to set boundaries and not feel so responsible and overwhelmed, their thinking becomes less confusing. Eventually they begin to make sense.

✓ **CLIENT'S REPEATING UNHEALTHY PATTERNS:** As clients share their story, it's helpful for them to have us identify unhealthy patterns that we see. This clarification can bring on an "ah-ha" moment for them. Many codependents are completely unaware that some of their dysfunctional thoughts, feelings, and behaviors are unhealthy and detrimental to their relationships and themselves. For example, a wife may report that she is in charge of making appointments for her husband rather than having him take care of his own responsibilities. For others, they may have gotten into financial difficulty to keep their partner happy, spending money they really didn't have or want to spend. Highlighting these enabling behaviors will provide teaching for the client about <u>choosing</u> what they want to do for others. It's okay to be helpful and caring toward others, but not at the expense of themselves.

• REDIRECT THE CLIENT'S FOCUS FROM OTHERS TO SELF

When codependents come into counseling as new clients, you will find that they are often hyper-focused on someone in their life. They start the counseling process by asking a lot of questions about their loved ones, rather than talking about themselves. They want to learn how to make those people change and do what they've asked them to do. Of course, this causes a lot of conflict.

Their questions are, in a positive way, a chance for the individual to better understand addiction, neglect and family-of-origin or mental health issues. However, their focus on others becomes so much a part of their day-to-day living that they have no idea what they feel or what they want. And this curiosity about changing others can derail the counseling process.

Be highly attuned to this dynamic. If you find that you are supporting the client by answering all the questions they have about another person, you are going in the wrong direction. Therapists not trained in working with codependency can get tripped up here. You may feel stuck, as does the client. You may be trying to help them determine what diagnosis you would suggest for their loved one. But know that it's a diversion of the client's from focusing on themselves. They want to understand the other person's problems so they can help them change. Learning to let go of others and allowing them to make decisions for themselves is a very difficult concept to learn. Keep at it!

It will be important for you to help redirect their focus on themselves. For example, ask them how they feel about a particular situation that might include their loved one. "How are you doing with all this?" is a good question. "What emotions come up for you?" Help them identify feelings around the issues they are bringing up.

If the session is more about someone else, you can also redirect the client in this way, "We're talking more about your partner than we are talking about you. Let's get back to your feelings now." I will remind them, "You can't change the other person. You can't control them or make them do what you want them to do. So let's focus on the person you can control...you."

Taking care of others, worrying about others, keeping tabs on others causes the client to feel exhausted. If you hear your client talk about feeling overwhelmed...this can be a red flag!

• MOVE CLIENTS FROM DENIAL TO AWARENESS

No one can change their life without first having awareness that a problem exists. For codependent people, they have lived in denial as a way to feel safe and avoid the issues. We all understand that denial is a great place to live because we don't have to make decisions or admit that there is a problem.

Some people don't want to admit that they have problems either individually or in their relationships. They have learned to ignore the issues and "stuff" the feelings of the dysfunction going on around them. Admitting the problems the client is facing can be terrifying for them. If they admit their husband is mentally ill, they may be afraid that they have to "do" something, i.e. leave the marriage. Admitting to having other difficulties may put them in a position of being judged by others. For example, if a client's child has gotten into trouble, the parents may feel they have failed in their parenting and this shame can keep them in denial.

Codependents have lived with difficult dysfunction for a long time and they can't bear it any longer. Usually they are in love with someone with an addiction, (work, drugs, alcohol, sex, etc.) or they have been a caregiver for so long they've lost their own identity and tried for years to change their situation, but to no avail. They may have tried to control or change the other person and have only felt frustrated, angry, powerless, and hopeless.

Breaking free from denial can be very challenging and it will be important for clinicians to not force them into reality. This can bring on more shame and cause the client to become defensive and protective of themselves. When the clients don't feel safe, they will discontinue therapy.

Much like addiction, denial is prevalent in codependency.

HOW CAN WE HELP? I've found psycho-education as a great way to ease into the client's denial. I suggest reading books and handouts, and I offer in-session training during our counseling. See the resource list at the end of the book for helpful reading materials. Giving the client the knowledge about this disorder can help them feel more in control of themselves and break down the walls of denial. This is a great start and helps them understand the issue and their reactions to the dysfunction.

In AA, addicts learn about their inner circle. Inside the inner circle are the coping strategies they have utilized to manage life. These strategies, however, are self-harming and hurt others in the mix. For example, clients may be struggling with their marriage and they have found that dealing with their problems was too difficult so they learned to self-medicate in some way. Addicts choose alcohol, sex, work, etc. Codependents choose controlling others, anger, abuse and denial. (See page 35 for a list of typical poor coping strategies.) As they realize their denial was a way to keep them safe (because admitting the problem was too difficult for them), we can discuss together other options of coping.

We have to work very diligently to focus on the client and not on the other people in their life. It's critical to deal with the denial, and help the client understand the issues they have been living with and not let those little denial statements go unanswered such as "It's not that bad," "I can handle it," or "I don't want to hurt him." Identify, identify, identify. But do so with empathy, education and planning together.

- ## DEAL WITH CONTROL ISSUES

Because we see control as such an issue in codependent relationships, we need to help the client understand what is and is not under their control. Facing codependency and focusing on the self, the codependent must learn to identify feelings, acknowledge wants and desires, understand healthy boundaries, and realize what they have control over.

For some, control has served them well in their life. They look really put together when they are in control and can organize events, projects, etc. But what is not seen by an outsider is the anxiety and fear that some of these people live with 24/7. Taking control may feel as though it takes care of the anxiety (and it does alleviate anxiety at times), but it really covers up the anxiousness the individual is actually feeling. The basis of anxiety is really not addressed and resolved, just simply covered up and managed for a time by controlling behaviors.

People with these issues often have others in their life who feel angry and frustrated with them because they have such a "controlling nature." This trait feels obnoxious, overbearing, and just plain annoying. People don't like others who try to control them and may avoid them because they are so hard to be around. Since this comes from a fear-based belief system, teaching strategies to manage their anxiety will help with their control issues.

One thing we want our clients to understand is how their control has intensified the unhealthy situation. By stepping in and taking care of someone else's responsibility only keeps the individual who is truly responsible for themselves reliant on the codependent and ultimately irresponsible. The codependent may make excuses such as, "I was only trying to help," or "If I don't do it, it won't get done," or "I'm more responsible than he/she is, so I'll take charge of it." This only leaves the codependent more exhausted and resentful and the loved one reliant on others and irresponsible for their own behavior and life.

HOW CAN WE HELP? Cermak identifies a stage of recovery from codependency as Re-Identification Stage (Stage II). Here, the individual has to re-identify to themselves who they are. For many it comes at a time when their life feels really out of control, or their pain is undeniably difficult. It's much like the alcoholic who "hits bottom." The codependent realizes they have no control over the person they are concerned with, and they have come to a place of complete despair. Although very painful for the client, as a therapist, this is a great step forward. Their awareness of their inability to keep it all together is a starting point for recovery from codependency, so celebrate this benchmark.

The second part of the Re-Identification Stage (Stage II), according to Cermak, involves the acceptance of their limitations. After codependents have realized they are powerless in the situation, that their strategies to make their relationship work haven't helped, then they can learn to accept their limitations. For some, they feel relief...relief that they haven't failed and relief that it's not their fault. But for some, if they don't get through this stage, they can fall into the "victim" role, or the "martyr" role. So it's important to get through this second phase.

In Cermak's Core Issues Stage (Stage III), the codependent can look at the issues of independence and autonomy. Along with understanding boundaries, the codependent can see that their wishes for their loved one or their hope for their family may truly be out of their hands. Cermak suggests that "the Core Issues Stage, then, is one of detaching oneself from the struggles of one's life - struggles which exist because of prideful and willful efforts to control those things which are beyond one's power to control." (pg. 75)

At Stage IV, the Re-Integration Stage from Cermak's book, after letting go of their power over others, codependent people must regain the power over themselves. As the codependent's self worth increases and they learn to accept themselves for who they are, quirks and all (much like their acceptance of their loved one), they now can learn to do things for themselves, rather than feeling the right to control others.

As Cermak suggests, "how does one achieve integrity? He says with awareness, not denial; honesty, not secrecy; and a conscious connection with God, not arrogance. All of which can be progressively cultivated." (pg. 76)

I will talk about and explore the issue of anxiety. Where do they notice their anxiety? When do they notice it? As they become more aware of the anxiety they hold, they will be able to look at the control issues and see how anxiety and control work together. We explore situations in which they took control (which was not appreciated by the people in their lives) and discuss what would have happened had they not taken control? What other options would they have had when feeling anxious? We then work on deep breathing, relaxation and a "safe place" as a way to alleviate anxiety which in turn will help with trying to control people and situations (see pages 161-163).

As an EMDR certified therapist, I would also work with them using EMDR strategies to identify where the control issues may have begun. At what age? What were the situations going on in their life where they felt they had to take control? What would it say about them if they didn't have control? They're worthless? They're unsafe? Where in their bodies do they feel the anxiety? There may be a variety of negative cognitions they would claim they have experienced in their life, so take time to address those negative thoughts.

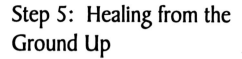

Step 5: Healing from the Ground Up

• ADDRESS FAMILY-OF-ORIGIN ISSUES

As a family therapist, I'm always interested in finding out about the family system in which the client grew up. I believe that the issues that arise for a client today are impacted by historical events. In other words, if a client has intense feelings about an event happening now, and we explore their history and go back in time, they can usually recall a situation in their past where they felt the same way as they feel in the present.

People struggling with codependency have had problems in their family system during their growing-up years. Many people who have grown up in alcoholic families or chronically ill families have either learned to be very responsible by taking care of their parents rather than themselves, or have been totally detached and disconnected from their family. Perhaps they were responsible for raising their siblings or were themselves raised by an older brother or sister. It's important to understand these dynamics by exploring the client's family of origin and processing through these events to teach them new ways of relating to others now as adults.

By understanding the family history, you can help your clients first understand and be aware of the unhealthy coping strategies they've learned. It will then be beneficial to delve into and get healing from those old wounds.

As a young wife, I didn't realize how much baggage I brought into my marriage. I didn't understand the concept of codependency and I thought I was doing great. I was happy, I was invested in my family by raising my three kids, and life was good. Then over time as I got tired and felt burdened with responsibility (I felt I was taking care of everything, the house, the yard, the kids, school and bills) it only left me angry and resentful. I thought I was doing what a good wife was supposed to do but I didn't like all of the responsibility.

I realize now that I learned to be overly responsible and learned to care for others rather than myself. As I gained insight and understanding through my counseling process (along with healing the wounds of abuse) and began setting boundaries, asking for what I needed (after much time figuring out what I did need), and began the journey of recovery from codependency, only then did I start to feel satisfied and happy in my life.

This process was also helpful in understanding and managing my emotions that felt out of control at times. I would have high anxiety, anger and resentment and didn't know how to manage those emotions. Healing from codependency brought peace into my life along with healthier relationships, for which I am so grateful!

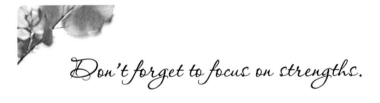

Don't forget to focus on strengths.

As I did my counseling, I wish I had understood that my parents did the best they could. However, I did blame them and did sever my relationship with my mother for one year (my father had died years before). I believe it's important to help clients understand that as humans, we all make mistakes. Our parents made mistakes and we, as parents, have made our share of mistakes as well. I only wish during my own counseling we would have spent some time exploring what good I did get from my family. I want to help clients put value on the positive aspects of their family system as well as look at the negative or difficulty they experienced growing up. Finding the balance, I believe, is important for all clients.

HOW CAN WE HELP? There are two ways I have worked with clients to understand their family of origin and helped them process through those issues. The first is the genogram. By drawing a picture of the family system and exploring the dynamics, abuse issues, strained relationships, and the wounds that result from the dysfunction, both you and the client can see patterns and reasons for the problems and you can also build on the family strengths.

The second exercise that I've found helpful for clients to understand their family system and their own wounds is called the Life Development Project (it's also called "The Egg" and can be found on page 144). This project is done by the client at home to identify and draw out their memories of growing up. It looks at the positive and the negative aspects of their family. I encourage clients to take their time while doing the project, to just let the memories come, by relaxing into the exercise and know that whatever comes to mind is what is meant to be worked on at this point. I also ask that they include their sexual history, which for some, may be the first time they've discussed this with anyone else. They will find that once they get started, they will begin to remember more and more.

In each corner of the page they are drawing, they are asked to recall the rules of the family and write those rules down, both spoken and unspoken, then the roles of each family member. In the bottom two corners, they are asked to write the traits for mom on one side and the traits for dad on the other side. If they had other caregivers such as a step parent, grandparent, foster or adoptive parents, include them as well. The four corners of the "egg" are to be written and the memories inside the "egg" are drawn.

In each cell of the "egg" they are asked to draw pictures. "I can't draw," is the typical response I get from my clients. I remind them that most people are not great artists and to just notice their anxiety about art and know that there is no right or wrong way to do this. Drawing helps get to the unconscious, so it's preferred rather than writing words.

Have them start with their earliest memory for the first cell and continue up through the years with each cell and each memory. Include monumental events, positive and negative, such as having a child, the death of a parent, etc. If they need help remembering what each drawing is, I encourage them to have a "cheat-sheet" with a list describing each cell.

When they return the next week, we start going over the exercise. I will encourage them to start with the corners of their "egg" and talk about the roles and rules they grew up with, along with the traits of their parents. As you review the cells of their "egg", take time to ask questions and help the client talk about and express the emotions as they go over their memories. You will notice that clients may want to quickly skip over events, much like reporting, but encourage them to slow down and talk about everything. (You may be dealing with shame, so don't ignore their reluctance.) You can take your time to also teach them about emotions by offering ideas about how you might feel if you'd had a similar experience. As you listen and acknowledge their story, they will feel heard and understood which is very therapeutic.

Some of the clients' experiences have caused feelings of shame and embarrassment and because of those emotions, they may never have shared these events with anyone. It will be important for the therapist to not be shocked by any aspect of their story. Acknowledge their experience, explore more, and thank them for being honest because you understand how difficult it might have been for them to be open with you.

This project is an effective way to dig into troubling events very quickly. Often clients will be embarrassed about some of their memories and for many, having the therapist normalize some of their experiences alleviates the guilt, shame or remorse. The telling of their story to a non-judgmental person helps them open up and be more honest and when we listen without critique, their shame will diminish.

This process of completing the "egg" can take several sessions and I've done it in small pieces over several weeks of counseling. However you choose to work through this project, just be sure to complete it at some point and do what you do best...acknowledge, normalize, listen, encourage, process and provide healing for their wounds.

Life Development Project
(The Egg)

This project is helpful in identifying patterns of behaviors across an individual's life span. It is also helpful in identifying how family of origin contributed to patterns of behavior, feelings or thoughts. By identifying and understanding life development patterns, areas of life that are problematic are revealed and focus of work can be clarified, leading to opportunities for change to occur. See the next page for the drawing.

- Find a large sheet of art paper. Markers or any writing utensil is acceptable.
- On the art paper, draw a large oval that takes up most of the sheet.
- Outside of the oval and at the bottom of the page, write your mother's positive and negative characteristics on one side and your father's positive and negative characteristics on the other side. Approximately 5-10 traits are sufficient. Include other caregivers who were also influential.
- On the upper corners of the sheet, outside the oval, list your family rules, both spoken and unspoken, and list your family members' roles.
- Think of events in your life that were significant, positive, painful, embarrassing, or when you felt let down. Starting with the earliest memory from childhood, draw a symbol for each item and separate it by a small curve. Use pictures to identify those experiences. Recent memories should be near the top and early memories toward the bottom of the "egg". Work slowly. This project should take some time.

Family Rules (i.e. get your work done before play; keep dad happy at all costs; appreciate what you have (little children are starving in other countries); don't rock the boat. etc.)

Family Roles (i.e. hero, princess, clown, scapegoat, doer, enabler, care-taker, saint, etc.)

Fill in your "egg" with positive and negative events from your life, starting with your earliest memories. Add a new "half moon" for each event. Draw a picture in the "half moon" to symbolize the event. Listen to your instincts as to what to include. Think about school, family, church, friends, extra-curricular activities, and sexual experiences.

Mother's Traits
(positive & negative)

Father's Traits
(positive & negative)

- ## BUILD SELF-ESTEEM

Codependency breeds poor self-esteem. Low self-esteem develops from criticism and abuse in the family system. This dysfunction permeates the children like a plague and follows them into adulthood. Sometimes if the parents think less of themselves and also have poor self-esteem, the children can take on those characteristics and live life with a feeling of "less-than."

However, some children can go toward the other extreme and become grandiose and arrogant, using the criticism and abuse they have received to be critical, self-righteous and judging of others. This dysfunctional family system teaches children that they are better than others. Or if an individual has experienced sexual abuse at the hands of a trusted adult, they begin feeling superior or "special" which can be a set-up for thinking others are "less-than" they are. Self-righteous thinking and behaving evolves and this false sense of power or grandiosity causes major adult relationship issues and unhappiness.

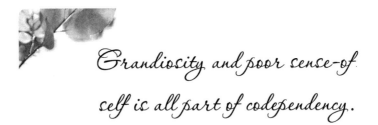

Grandiosity and poor sense-of self is all part of codependency.

Pia Mellody identifies "other esteem" as a fragile outlook on self. What she is saying is that some individuals base their worth on what others think of them, such as: how they look, how much money they make, who they know, what kind of car, house or job they have, how well their children behave and perform, how attractive their spouse is, what degrees they have earned, etc. This is a fragile outlook because if we make any mistakes or our loved ones make mistakes, our esteem can crumble and shame can escalate. The power of another's perspective can take control of the individual, rather than the person having control of themselves.

HOW CAN WE HELP? Helping to build your client's self-esteem requires a lot of patience and your ability to be present, accepting, and providing healthy alternatives. As clients learn new coping strategies to deal with dysfunctional situations, learn healthy boundaries and understand what it means to be authentic and accepting of themselves, their esteem will build. In the process they may realize that they have said "No" to someone and it went over very well, or chose not to get involved in an obligation where they normally may have done so. All of these successes will build their self-esteem. As you normalize their experiences and their approaches to situations, your clients will begin to feel proud of themselves and realize how strong and competent they really are.

Another strategy I use to build self-esteem involves a simple homework assignment. I ask the client to be aware of how they respond to positive reinforcement from others. I ask them to notice compliments from others, such as acknowledgement about positive changes they have made, compliments about their actions, their looks, etc. I encourage them to respond with "Thank You." They are to give no excuses, no pushing the compliment away, just say "Thank You." This is very difficult for many people to do. But it is do-able and will help them take in positive feedback that is normally pushed away.

Building self-esteem will be a part of all your therapy, and know that the client's confidence will rise as you encourage, praise, and help identify areas of their life where they've grown. I would encourage reassessing how the counseling process is going for them; in fact, I suggest reviewing it every five to six weeks. As you both identify the changes they have made and share with them the positive strides they have accomplished, it's very rewarding for everyone. It's rewarding as a therapist to see the client blossom into a confident and independent person, and the clients will be pleased with the positive experiences and successes they realize they have experienced.

- ## IDENTIFY & SET HEALTHY BOUNDARIES

Many unhealthy families either have no boundaries at all or rigid boundaries that constrain the family system. If a client has experienced abuse, the boundaries in their family are non-existent and anyone is welcome in, even if those people are abusive and unhealthy. Another unhealthy extreme includes families who have very rigid boundaries where new-comers or in-laws coming into the family are rejected, excluded and not accepted, no matter how hard they try. Healthy boundaries fluctuate and move depending on who or what wants to infiltrate the family system.

Beattie identifies dysfunctional boundaries as those that violate others, or others violating ours. They are the definition of our personal space (and those that violate that space are called abusers or perpetrators). If individuals don't have good self-esteem, they may allow others to abuse them causing victimization.

Often children who are abused, whether physically, emotionally, sexually, or verbally, have not had people to protect them and shown them how, or given them permission, to say "No" if they feel someone is infiltrating their space. Unfortunately, these individuals tend to get victimized again and again throughout their lives.

Beattie identifies four kinds of boundary impairments. The first is *no boundary* at all. These people have no sense or are cognitively unaware of being abused or of abusing others. They are unaware that they violated others' boundaries or that other people violated their own boundaries.

Some families may have had one parent as the abuser and the other parent too intimidated to protect the child, or themselves. Both of these parents did not learn what healthy touch and words were and didn't know how to set those limits.

BEATTIE'S BOUNDARY IMPAIRMENTS

1. No boundary at all
2. Damaged boundaries
3. Walls instead of boundaries
4. Unpredictable boundaries

The second boundary impairment includes *damaged boundaries.* These individuals can, at times, say "No" to certain individuals, set limits, or take care of themselves, and for others they feel powerless and have difficulty saying "No" to authority figures, such as parents or bosses. These individuals struggle with setting boundaries when they are stressed, tired or feeling weak. These people may step in where they are not wanted and they may try to control a situation when their anxiety gets high, while at other times, they are able to step away and keep appropriate limits.

The third boundary impairment includes *walls instead of boundaries.* These people have difficulty letting others into their lives emotionally and physically. Some exhibit anger and their anger has worked well as a way to keep people at arm's length. Other people use a "wall of fear," (Beattie, pg. 16) and retreat from relationships because they are so frightened. Many of these people seem quiet and simply observe life around them. Because these clients are so fear-based, you as their therapist may feel concerned they will fall apart or explode.

And then there are those individuals who can *maneuver between no boundaries and walled off boundaries.* This can feel confusing for the people around them because it's unpredictable. And as an outsider they may feel close to someone because they are sharing more than they may otherwise, but then as you try to get close emotionally, they back off and wall up. It's a crazy dance and a difficult relationship in which to get close.

Our job as therapists is to encourage clients to take risks. Setting boundaries can be very risky and in some families cause relationships to be destroyed. A parent who is, for the first time, hearing "No" from their child (even when the child is an adult), may respond by disowning their child. The person with whom the client is trying to set the boundary may lash out with anger, resentment, and potentially physical, emotional, verbal, or sexual abuse. In these cases, it will be important to have a plan and be prepared with a strategy for the client to protect themselves.

HOW CAN WE HELP? Here are several ideas to consider:

✓ Planning is essential for the client so they are prepared for whatever reaction their loved one may have. If there is a concern for physical abuse, talk in your session about strategies of presenting their boundaries. What this means is practicing (using a script if necessary) having the conversation with their loved one. It may even be important to identify potential shelters if they are in imminent danger. Their safety is paramount, so evaluate if there is abuse in this situation and consider all scenarios as it's better to plan for the worst. Remember to encourage them to stay strong.

✓ The fear many codependent people feel will need to be addressed with new cognitive behavioral strategies, gently reminding them that these changes, or "adjustments," are important steps to healthy living. You, as the therapist, will be their biggest encourager and can help them process through the rejection, anger and other emotions coming from the person with whom they've set the boundary. It's tough and scary for the client, so encourage, encourage, encourage.

✓ Because setting boundaries can be so difficult, it's important for the client to have a support system. Help your clients identify the supportive, safe people they have in their lives, or if they lack support, encourage them to build a network of friends they can trust. Cloud and Townsend encourage this step because trying these new strategies can be challenging without help. Also, most everyone will feel a sense of guilt as they set boundaries and they will need others to walk alongside them as they learn to master this new skill.

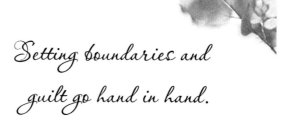

Setting boundaries and guilt go hand in hand.

✓ When you are helping an individual set boundaries start small. For example, help them start with setting their own boundary by saying, "No" to a food craving, or saying, "No" to a thought. As they become more and more comfortable, begin with someone other than a family member as starting with less intense relationships can be less threatening. Gradually work toward setting boundaries with family members and remind the client that feeling guilt and concern for their loved ones will probably come up. Remind them it's normal but continue setting limits in spite of the guilt.

Awareness of healthy living, having safe people (like you as their therapist) surrounding them and offering encouragement for taking risks are all important as well as helping them identify their progress, celebrating their successes, and supporting their needs when dealing with boundary setting and codependency.

I will outline for you three strategies I use around boundary setting that I have found helpful and successful. Initially, I believe psycho-education will be helpful to understand the issue. So I have used the following diagram as a teaching tool. I honestly can't recall where this diagram came from as I'd like to give the person the credit they deserve. But it's been a very helpful visual tool I've used with many clients and is a way to help them understand family boundaries.

Family System Boundaries Diagram

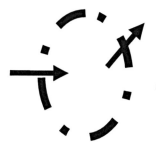

This family system is too open where anyone can come and go, even unsafe, abusive people. Here members may exit the family with no connections or will have broken relationships.

This family system is too closed where few people can enter. Here families are enmeshed with little outside influence.

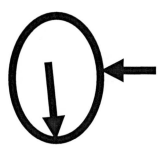

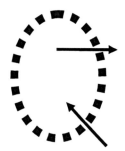

This family system is somewhat open and flexible, where people are invited in and included. Here members are healthy and understand and honor clear, appropriate boundaries.

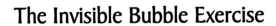

The Invisible Bubble Exercise

Next, this strategy is something I use often with my clients when dealing with verbal/emotional abuse. I ask them to think about an imaginary bubble surrounding them when they talk with their loved one(s), imagining all the words, accusations, and negativity bouncing off the invisible bubble without allowing the negativity "in." In other words, I help them visualize the words being directed at the bubble and they don't penetrate their heart. I found it helpful for me as I was learning boundary strategies. I'm amazed at how powerful imagination can be to help clients with their trauma. As they imagine these new ways of doing things, they are "remapping" their brain. Making a new outcome can bring all the relief they need.

And thirdly, the following activity called The Hoops Exercise is a very practical and visually helpful tool for clients as you discuss boundaries. Clients love it because it provides them a language to talk with others (i.e. "Please stay out of my hoop.") They can visualize this in their minds to remind themselves to "stay in their own hoop." Try this with your clients. I think you will see a positive and grateful response.

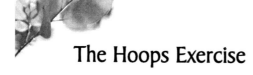

The Hoops Exercise

Place two hula hoops on the floor. Standing in one, explain that this is their hoop and it contains their thoughts, feelings, behaviors, beliefs, hopes, dreams, body, desires, decisions, family system, responsibilities, etc. All of these belong to them and are under their control. The client is truly living in their own hoop when they know what they like and don't like, and make decisions for themselves based on their needs and desires and no one else's.

The second hoop is for their loved one. In this hoop are the same things as what is in their own hoop: hopes, dreams, desires, etc. Ideally we take care of our own hoop and don't invade the other's hoop. Unfortunately, this is oftentimes not the case.

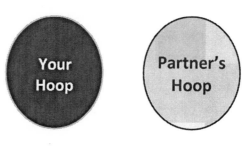

Now when codependents are controlling others by giving them their opinions, or telling them what they "should" do, they are completely out of their hoop and into their loved one's. So, where does their partner go? They leave their hoop and disengage, get angry and frustrated with the codependent and detach. Who is taking care of the codependent's hoop? No one. It's empty, much like how the codependent feels, with no one understanding their wants and needs. The codependent person is strictly focused on what the other person "should" do or "should" be feeling.

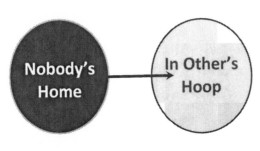

No one likes to have others control them and they will avoid people who are trying to do so. As the loved one moves out of their hoop because the codependent person is there running the show, the loved one has to go somewhere. Where do you suppose they go? They engage in unhealthy coping strategies such as drug or alcohol abuse, workaholism, sex addiction, and outside relationships. Although it's not the codependent's responsibility to keep their loved one from choosing these negative coping strategies, it's certainly makes sense that poor choices are made when someone is trying to control the other person.

When people abandon their hoop (or focus on others), intimacy is non-existent and the codependent has no awareness or understanding of their own wants and needs. Their entire focus is on the other person, leaving the codependent powerless and hopeless, which only makes them try even harder to get closer to their loved one. We then have what is called the "pursuer-distancer" behavior. The more the codependent pursues, the more the loved one distances themselves from that person.

When I talk with clients about their marriage, I will have a third hoop on the floor for the "marriage" hoop. Following are the typical relationship stages couples go through. It's a great teaching for couple's to understand the issue of boundaries.

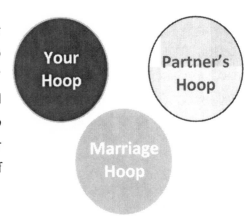

✓ **AUTONOMOUS STAGE** - (Each person is in their own hoop and the relationship hoop is empty). This stage is about the person's individuality, their thoughts, feelings, actions, beliefs, values, experiences, all parts of the individual. This is prior to meeting one another. However, I also see individuals who have left a marriage want to go back to this stage to figure out who they are.

✓ **INFATUATION STAGE** - (Both people are in the couple's hoop). The couple have met one another and they are very focused on the relationship and have forgotten about their own hoop. Often peoples' brains don't work as well and they also don't see one another's faults at this stage. It's bliss. But then after the Infatuation Stage, someone shifts and moves back into their "normal" life and back into their hoop (for example, focusing back on self/work/other responsibilities). The tough part of this stage is that one person may not be ready to move back into their Autonomous Stage and may feel abandoned or left behind. Or possibly someone has gone back to their old way of living and/or their negative coping strategies (i.e., back to alcohol, drugs, work, whatever they choose to cope negatively, etc.)

✓ **DIFFERENTIATION STAGE** - (Both people go back to their individual hoop.) At this stage, each individual is learning several things such as:

o How to become their own person in the relationship and how that works.

o To fix the relationship one person may move closer to the other person in his/her hoop. Here, we as therapists may see blaming, anger, criticism, wanting the other person to change. As they feel the other person pull away, they may move closer, clinging, holding on to the other in desperation.

o As they learn to cope outside of their hoop, they could turn to their negative coping strategies (alcohol, drugs, others) that can be hurtful to them, their partner and their relationship.

o They may have trouble with differentiation and it can be very hard to leave the other's hoop due to fear of abandonment, anxiety and other emotions.

o Safety is also an issue for them in their relationship. When they don't feel safe and secure in the relationship, it's very difficult to leave the other's hoop.

✓ **RECOVERY STAGE** - (Both individuals are in their own hoop.) The couple may be emotionally and physically separate as they sort through the relationship issues. An individual can have one foot in the hoop and one foot out. One person may have more difficulty than the other with the Recovery Stage if they've had trauma in their life and are using negative coping skills. This stage can take a long time as each person learns to heal and grow.

✓ **INTERDEPENDENCE STAGE** - (One foot is in their own hoop and one foot is in the marriage hoop.) Here the couple is choosing the relationship out of desire, rather than out of neediness. This is a high stage of development. Some can put more emphasis in their marriage rather than their own hoop when they are healthy and clear about their own boundaries, wants and needs.

When people stay in their own hoop, it means that they are aware of who they are. Also, they are observant of things and people around them, and they're present. They understand healthy relationships and respond to their world from their "Wise Chair."

You can add your own ideas in this hoops exercise to fit your clients. Encourage the client to step into the hoops and talk about how it feels to be inside their own and then how it feels to be in the partner's hoop. Explore this idea in depth, taking some time and going over it again and again as boundary issues arise throughout the counseling process.

I have found this exercise so helpful in alleviating shame because as I ask, "What hoop are you in?" Typically the client laughs instead of feeling shame about their mistakes. It's also an easy concept for the clients to share with their loved ones by offering their family a language which allows everyone to talk openly about caring for themselves.

This exercise was introduced to me by Debbie Laaser while working with women who were in sexually addicted relationships. The concept of boundaries is often difficult for people to understand and this hula hoop exercise allows the clients to grasp it easily. I use it with all my clients, individually and in couple's sessions. For more information and a complete demonstration, see Faithfulandtrue.com for e-product and full demonstration.

• ADDRESS BODY RESPONSES

I always encourage my clients to notice their body. Where do they feel tension, hot, cold, pain, or pressure? Often their body can be telling them things their mind hasn't registered yet. They just need to learn to listen as it can tell them what their feeling by focusing on their body. For those individuals with anxiety, their stomach may be upset, their gastrointestinal tract is not working properly, they feel light-headed, or have tingling in their hands or feet, and racing heart and racing thoughts. For others, they have pressure or tension in their throat which can be indicative of the inability or unwillingness to talk or speak up.

I have found the book, *You Can Heal Your Life* by Louise Hay to be very helpful. She talks about the body and explains, in easy-to-understand detail, how certain symptoms can be indicative of emotions and beliefs. It's been a good resource guide that I refer to in the session to read to clients what their bodies may be trying to tell them. As I was doing work with a client recently, we were talking about his family history and he noticed pain and pressure behind his eyes. According to Ms. Hay's book, this indicated he didn't want to look back at his past. When I asked if that seemed to fit, he was amazed at how accurate it was. As much as he wanted to get healthier, his subconscious said, "Don't look back." This new insight offers the codependent person a chance to focus on unconscious beliefs in the counseling process.

Our body tells us what we are experiencing, so help clients learn to listen.

Often people who have experienced trauma or constant chaos in their lives (and their focus has had to be outside of themselves), learning to listen to their body's responses is a very difficult task. Many times trauma in early childhood can get "stuck" in the body memories, so it's important to identify and acknowledge their symptoms and encourage them to talk about what those symptoms are trying to convey. They can become extremely ill because they have ignored these signals too long and developed ulcers, cancer, chronic pain, auto-immune diseases and other devastating illnesses. Help the client address their physical symptoms and learn to trust their instincts. As they become better able to do this, they will be able to determine what desires need to be met and what faulty beliefs need to be addressed.

HOW CAN WE HELP?   Initially, I encourage clients to talk with their doctor and be sure there are no physical conditions that need to be addressed and treated. If they are healthy, I will suggest getting a massage and other holistic treatments, such as acupuncture, chiropractic and others that can be healing. I have also found EMDR to be a help tool to address bodily reactions.   Encourage your clients to take care of their physical symptoms and listen to what their body is trying to tell them.   The strategies I have also used in the counseling office include deep breathing, relaxation and visualization.

Deep Breathing Exercise

I teach the client how to breathe deeply by asking them to breathe down to their abdomen, allowing their stomach to "puff out."   Take their breath in through their nose, hold it for a few seconds and then exhale through their mouth, slowly, as though they are blowing through a straw. With each breath I ask them to notice their body, focusing on several muscle groups such as the shoulders, back, neck, abdomen, relaxing each muscle where the tension resides. Practicing this many times during the week can be helpful in acquiring skills to relaxation.

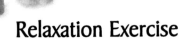

Relaxation Exercise

After learning the breathing exercise, I ask them to close their eyes and as a means to get to know their body better, I walk them through a tensing and relaxing of each muscle group from their head to their toes. They will become more aware of their body and the tension it holds and will be more attentive of their body cues.

As you know, take your time with the relaxation, talking softly and slowly to allow the client to relax even deeper.

1. Start with your head and tense the muscles of your forehead and scalp by raising your eyebrows upward, hold for three seconds, then let go and relax.

2. Now focus on your eyelids, tightening and squeezing them shut three seconds, then let go.

3. Move on to the cheeks, smile big and hold the muscles tense three seconds, then release. Notice the difference between the tight and relaxed muscles.

4. Move to the jaw muscles and clench your teeth together, hold three seconds and release.

5. For the neck and shoulders, lift your shoulders up toward your ears, hold the tension three seconds and release.

6. Now, curl your fingers making a fist, bend your arms at the elbow and bring your hands up toward the shoulders, hold and release.

7. For the scapulas (back bones in upper back), try to touch your elbows behind your back, hold three seconds and release.

8. For the chest and upper back, imagine a 12-in rubber band around your chest and suck your chest in toward your spine, hold and release.

9. For the abdomen, suck in your stomach and push it toward your spine, hold and release.

10. Tighten the gluteus muscles and hips, hold and release.

11. For your thighs, squeeze your knees together, hold and release.

12. For your calves, stretch the calves by raising your feet toward the ceiling, hold and release.

13. For your toes, curl the toes under, hold and release.

I will often progress from the Relaxation Exercise directly into the Safe Place Exercise. The Safe Place is a strategy used in EMDR. This exercise is very helpful for clients as a place they can go in their mind if they need relief from the traumatic memories, negative thoughts, or difficult feelings they are experiencing. It's been so helpful that I use it with all my clients.

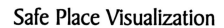

Safe Place Visualization

This exercise comes from the EMDR Protocol and I have found it very helpful for all clients, even if EMDR is not being used. This is how I direct the client:

Close your eyes if you are comfortable doing that (*or continue to keep your eyes closed after the Relaxation Exercise*). Take a moment and focus in on a place that feels safe and comforting to you. Take your time settling in somewhere and notice your body relaxing. *(Be quiet from time to time to let them get settled.)* Don't be surprised if you fluctuate from one spot to another, just notice that...eventually you will settle somewhere. Just take your time. Allow whatever comforting space comes to mind, and be gentle with yourself if you struggle.

Be aware of where you are...notice what you see. Be aware of the colors and textures surrounding you. *(Take your time and be quiet to allow them to focus.)* Consider, also, what you hear. Let your senses take in the calm and comforting sounds. Now realize what you feel on your skin. Perhaps it's a gentle breeze or cool air or the air is still. Just notice it and allow yourself to relax into those sensations. Also, be aware of what you smell. Allow those smells to continue to relax you even further.

Again, focus on your body in this safe, comforting place. Allow all your senses to be activated, taking it all in only to relax you. Be still for a moment and just be. *(Again, be quiet and let the client lean into this exercise even more.)*

(Take your time with this relaxation and safe place exercise and encourage the client to practice this at home several times a week. I encourage you to do this visualization often throughout the counseling process so it becomes second nature to the client.)

- **ADDRESS TRAUMA**

  Many children growing up in unhealthy homes have experienced some kind of abuse, trauma and/or neglect. A relationship between parental addiction and child abuse has been documented in a large proportion of child abuse and neglect cases. According to the National Association for Children of Alcoholics:

  ✓ Three of four (71.6%) child welfare professionals cite substance abuse as the top cause for the dramatic rise in child maltreatment since 1986.

✓ Most welfare professionals (79.6%) report that substance abuse causes or contributes to at least half of all cases of child maltreatment; 39.7% say it is a factor in over 75% of the cases.

✓ In a sample of parents who significantly abuse their children, alcohol abuse is specifically associated with physical abuse, while cocaine exhibits a specific relationship to sexual maltreatment.

✓ Children exposed prenatally to illicit drugs are 2 to 3 times more likely to be abused or neglected.

Unfortunately, if a parent is addicted or unavailable to their child for a variety of reasons (i.e., poor emotional intimacy skills), we know that those children grow up with insecure emotional attachments, difficulty with intimacy of all kinds, and other problems. We have to be ready to address those issues of trauma with the people coming in to see us for codependency.

When I was in my own counseling sessions, I believe my therapist was aware of my abuse long before I was. You see, my mind had repressed all my sexually abusive memories. However, I had glimpses of memories or snapshots, if you will, but I couldn't put the pieces together. Then at one particularly painful session, the trauma memories came up and my therapist was ready. It was a very painful part of my recovery and I'm so grateful that the memories did come so I could work on those abusive experiences. But it was extremely important that my therapist did not place any ideas of abuse in my mind. She never suggested it. She let it come up when the time was right and when I believed I was strong enough to handle it. So, be very careful. Don't suggest abuse, just wait for it to show up.

HOW CAN WE HELP? Listen attentively and if you hear things like "I don't remember much of my childhood" or, "What someone did to me was 'icky'," these are indications, but not certain signs, of abuse. Remember, just wait!

I have found EMDR to be a very effective treatment strategy for clients with abuse issues. I have used it for several years and a strategy in EMDR is to ask the client to "float back," in time to old abuses and while they "float back," other memories can be tapped and explored. It's a great tool. What I love about EMDR is that if the client feels flooded or overwhelmed, we visualize a safe and comforting place to relieve the flooding (See the Safe Place Exercise on page 163). Then, when the client is ready, we can return to the memories. But it's done slowly and at the client's pace which can help them learn to manage emotions more effectively.

PTSD and codependency can be very much intertwined and a good therapist will help unravel these issues at the client's pace. Much of the strategies used for PTSD, such as addressing emotions, validating experiences, managing the memories, dealing with the depression and anxiety, will all be helpful for codependency issues as well. The Life Development Project, or "The Egg," (see page 144) is a great way to reveal the trauma of a codependent's life. Take the time to explore the past and help the client heal those wounds.

For those people whose parents were unavailable due to chronic illness, addiction, mental health issues, and more, they may have not learned how to create positive emotional connections. Too many children have learned to live with loneliness, hopelessness, fear, and other problems and we see them in our office every day! Many codependents who acknowledge neglect may feel very loyal to their caregivers and not want to disparage them. Much like repressed memories, take it slow and remind the client that you are going back not to blame their parents, but simply to learn how the situation affected them and to work on healing those wounds. Their parents did the best they could and they have positive memories as well. Then, acknowledge those positive memories and good times and balance them with the more difficult or abusive experiences.

There is much more that's needed to deal with the trauma, as you know. This is just a quick overview of some of the issues you will come across in the counseling office. If you are not trained in a protocol that treats trauma, I would encourage you to get the training.

• DISCUSS SPIRITUAL RENEWAL

My healing from codependency was a fulfilling process and I believe part of what was important for me was reconnecting with my faith in Christ. I did, however, need to get through the painful aspects of my journey before I could allow my spirituality and faith in God to emerge. I have found that some of my clients need to go through the healing of their backgrounds as well before they come to reconciling their faith journey or spirituality.

I believe it's important for all therapists to be cognizant of each client's need and/or desire for a connection with God. As a Christian therapist, my goal is to offer hope even in situations that may seem overwhelming and hopeless. I'm always sensitive to each client's need for spiritual recovery and if it's important for the client, I'm happy to walk alongside them as they sort this out. If it's not important for the client, that's up to them.

I'm sure many other people have yearned for a spiritual relationship and wanted something that could fill the void in their soul. As therapists, we need to be ready and willing to help them explore the spiritual aspect of their lives.

Through the 12-Step programs, addressing the connection with a "Higher Power" is important in the healing journey. Some people have found this spiritual connection very calming and supportive and it's made a real difference in their lives. When they've learned to give up control to their spiritual being, they feel enormous relief and satisfaction. As people who have really only trusted in themselves, it's a giant step toward their recovery, and also a continual work in progress. Help your clients take the baby steps they need in order to determine their own spiritual journey, and we can walk alongside them on this healing path.

Healing the pain may need to happen before a spiritual connection can be made.

HOW CAN WE HELP? At the first session I will go over our intake form which asks clients about their religious or spiritual beliefs. I talk with each client about their faith in terms of whether or not it's an important part of their life and whether they'd like to explore their spirituality while in therapy. For many clients, spiritual questions will arise at one time or another. Because so many of my clients come from referrals from churches, this topic comes naturally for them. However, other clients may be opposed to spiritual exploration and we need to be respectful of their desires.

While discussing this aspect of their lives, we examine together the beliefs they acquired from their church and family. Some have had very positive experiences and feel connected to God; however, others have had little or no church education and/or faith encouragement. They may be ready to do that as part of their counseling and if so, be available to help them process.

I believe we all are spiritual beings and it's a part of the psyche that needs to be explored. Finding out what they learned as children will be helpful for them to determine for themselves what beliefs fit for their lives now and what don't fit. If they are feeling internal discord, take time to dig deeper. Addressing old, faulty thinking can be done with a variety of counseling techniques. I offer EMDR to my clients as they sort through those flawed beliefs. It's very interesting to see the transformation as they realize what feels right for them now.

Some clients have come into therapy looking for help in understanding the Bible and have had very deep spiritual questions. For example, when clients are questioning God and feeling confused or angry about their pain, these are questions we'll explore in the session; however, if they cannot get answers that satisfy them, I will often refer them to a pastor or spiritual advisor who can be of greater help.

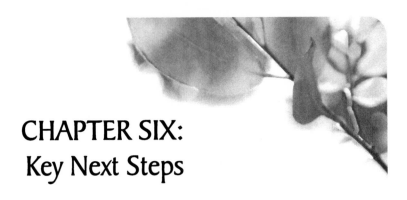

CHAPTER SIX:
Key Next Steps

The following information gives a broad overview of the key steps which have helped me, as well as many other friends, colleagues and clients address their codependency.

- ### 12-STEP GROUPS AND/OR AL-ANON

    I encourage everyone who is living with some kind of addiction, and/or sees their life as codependent, to get involved in an Al-anon or another 12-Step group. The encouragement and teaching from these groups is very helpful. It's a way to better understand addiction, codependency, and clients can learn how to can let go emotionally of their loved ones. Not only will participants begin looking at their own unhealthy behaviors, but they will realize that the addiction and dysfunction they grew up with was difficult. They will also learn to make changes for themselves and determine if they wish to live by their family's rules, values or behaviors.

    The support from these groups will provide the safety and encouragement all codependents need to make the changes they desire. As they work towards healthy living, they will need this support to set boundaries, detach with love, and gain the strength they need as they struggle with these life challenges. Codependency is about change and whenever we try to change our living situation, we can't do it without help and understanding from others.

- **INDIVIDUAL COUNSELING**

  Individual counseling is essential to get to the core of negative beliefs. Due to the impact codependency has on one's personal relationships, as well as to help a person to grow and recover, counseling is the best way to get to those deeper issues. Clients are surprised at how these earlier relationships are connected to their situation here and now. And to do that work, professional counseling is the way to reach the goals of serious recovery.

  I'm so grateful for the counseling I received. It was a very painful process and it was tough to face the abuse, addiction, and hurt I experienced. However, I was very determined to get healthy because I didn't want my children to go through the same dysfunction and I wanted to change our family dynamics. It can be done with perseverance and determination, along with outside support of friends and family.

  Through my individual, group and marital counseling, I have learned to love and accept myself and feel good about who I am. My relationships have grown much deeper because I can manage my emotions, thoughts and behaviors and I no longer fear emotional intimacy with others (well, it's a work in progress). This positive change has helped me to be authentic and I'm relieved to be myself...not someone I thought others wanted me to be. Because the shame has lifted, I have embraced my idiosyncrasies and can laugh at my mistakes. It wasn't until I cleaned out the old beliefs and dealt with the emotions, was I finally capable of having a deeper relationship with myself, with my loved ones and with God.

- **CHANGE IS GOOD**

  Change can be scary, but it is good. Actually, when working with clients, I try not to use the word change. It sounds daunting to them. And some clients are very clear they do not want to change. So I suggest using the word "adjust." It sounds less threatening and it feels like it's a choice and the individual has the power to make that choice for themselves.

If I hadn't followed God's prompting, if I hadn't been so unhappy and depressed and not sought help, I would have stayed stuck in my unhappiness. Yes, making changes (adjustments), or decisions that seemed beyond what I felt I could do (for example, deciding to go back to school with three little kids); only then did my life change for the better. I also believe God knew all along what He had planned for me which was to get healthy and then use my experiences to help others.

Support and encourage your clients to embrace change...not shy away from it. I've found that it's important to reassure them that change will not make them a different person but will allow them to be more open-minded and give them a freedom to love themselves. When they become more open-minded, their life can grow happily beyond their wildest dreams. There are no guarantees and nothing stays the same, so flexibility, even though it can cause some anxiety, is a much healthier way to relate to others and to live life.

- **FORGIVENESS**

  I believe part of the healing process is to help clients come to the stage of forgiveness. Many people are confused about what it means to forgive, however, and this can keep them stuck in their resentment, hurt and anger. It does not mean to condone someone's behavior or accept the unhealthy behaviors others may have perpetrated on them, but it's a personal process for the client. It's a chance to let go of the negative emotions and bitterness toward another that results from hurt.

  Many Christians feel they need to forgive sooner than is helpful for them. I believe forgiveness is the ultimate goal, but many who have had deep wounds need to process and "clean up" the pain of the perpetration, betrayal or hurt first. Pardoning too soon can only bury the pain deeper without getting processed and eliminated. Once the client has worked through the events and feels it's complete, the forgiveness piece will be more successful. I remind clients that this is not about condoning others unhealthy behavior but a gift for themselves to move on.

Forgiveness can relieve the *injured* party from the fury, depression, betrayal, and all the other emotions that go along with being victimized. We don't want our clients to stay victims. We want them to move forward. Encourage your clients to address the issue of forgiveness to lighten their heart and move on in their lives to bigger and better things.

I'm including a Forgiveness Exercise that I received many years ago at a workshop at Perspectives (which was a counseling center in Minnetonka, MN). Dr. Edith Staufer designed this process and I found much forgiveness by working through the steps. It may be something a person needs to do several times. So I hope you find it helpful for yourself and your clients.

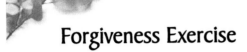

Forgiveness Exercise

1. Say to yourself, "I'm ready to stop suffering about what _____ (it might be yourself as well) has done (or not done).

2. Imagine that the person you are forgiving is in front of you (an empty chair or enrolling an object may help). Talk to them aloud about your hurt, anger, disappointment, etc.

3. Summarize your preferences about what "should" have occurred. Make this a positive statement, i.e. "I would have preferred that you had always been honest with me," or "I would prefer that you would agree to go to counseling with me." (Not "I wish you weren't such a jerk.")

4. Now, acknowledge: "But you're not like that and I will no longer suffer about it." Or, "But you didn't do those things; I now release those expectations. I choose to let it go and be free of it." It is important to state this as an act of will on your part.

5. Now, cancel those preferences/expectations one by one. "Therefore I cancel my expectation that you would always have been honest with me." "I cancel my expectation that you will go into counseling with me." Feel the power the word "cancel" has each time you say it.

6. Tell them, "...and I give you total responsibility for your actions (or attitudes)."

7. Focus your energy on God, imagining His presence and see Him as always protecting, loving, guiding and nurturing you all the days of your life. Contemplate the positive qualities of God until you feel those qualities flowing into you as healing love, peace, joy, acceptance, wisdom, compassion and understanding. Visualize and feel God's love cleansing and releasing all the expectations, demands and negativity.

8. When you feel clear and full of love, picture sending it to the person you are forgiving. Say to them, "I send you God's love, just as you are and as you have been; and I release you to God's care.

9. Think of a few things you like about them or a few things that are positive about your relationship.

10. Take an inventory of your body and emotions. What is different? Can you feel love for them? Do you feel a release? If you find you are still holding on to any demands or expectations, start from Step 1 again. If you are holding on, run it through the canceling process again. Or examine your willingness to be free and move on. Or there may be another related incident now resurfacing of which you were unaware which will need to be processed.

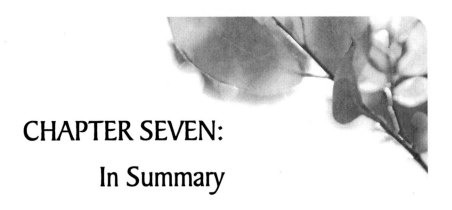

CHAPTER SEVEN:

In Summary

Counseling is not always pretty. It can be very painful and difficult. I learned new ways to think about things, redefined my values and beliefs for what fit for me and dealt with the pain of the dysfunction in my family. By taking time and focusing on my life, I realized I could have my own thoughts and beliefs and didn't need to believe necessarily what my family did. I learned that through the pain of the process, however, I was ultimately rewarded.

The help I received positively altered my relationship with my mother and I'm grateful for those last years we had together as equals. I learned to be myself, not be timid, threatened or intimidated by her and her anger, and I learned that her feelings, thoughts and desires belonged to her. By using the hula hoops to remind me of both our boundaries, I could let her have her feelings and I could be okay with hearing what she had to say. I didn't need to integrate her ideas into my life if it didn't fit for me. It was a great relief and ultimately diminished the anger and resentment I had towards her and other authority figures.

One of the most helpful tools I appreciated was learning to listen better to my loved ones...especially my husband. I had hoped and longed to know him better, but because I was often in his hoop, I was focused on changing him, educating him, counseling him and as you can imagine, it didn't go over very well. When I stopped trying to fix him and listen to his thoughts, ideas, values, and emotions, I learned to love him in a way I would never have been able to had I stayed stuck in my codependency. Relationships really can get better.

Because codependency causes dysfunctional relationships, many don't get to the real emotional and intimate part of their connections. I learned that I can be emotionally intimate with my loved ones and I don't need to be afraid. I have also chosen to surround myself with healthier relationships and work at fostering new, satisfying ones. I can now appreciate the friends and family I have and accept them for who they are, let them live their lives in the way they want to live and still love them.

As therapists, you will see codependency walk into your office often and now you have an organized strategy in which to help people. A word of caution, however; be careful that you are not in a codependent place yourself and wanting to take care of your clients. It's the client's responsibility to make those changes and pursue healthier relationships. And as I've said earlier, it's a very rewarding process for both the therapist and the client. To see people feel comfortable in their skin, make decisions for themselves, successfully set boundaries and grow is a wonderful thing to watch and experience. I hope something in my writing has struck a chord with you and if you've only learned one thing, that's good enough.

One last note...just being there for clients and providing a safe place in which they can talk and ultimately experience healing is therapeutic. I often hear from those people I supervise that they haven't felt they've done enough for their clients or haven't done enough "therapy" to help them. I tell them that their care, compassion and empathetic listening ear is powerful. For many codependents, they may never have experienced anyone who provided that for them in their lives. Let them feel your love and concern, guide them in their new journey, and walk alongside them as they enter their pain and you will have done enough.

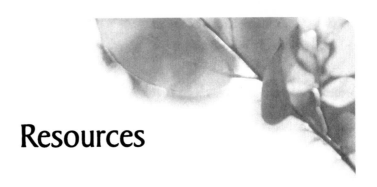

Resources

1. *One Day at a Time in Al-Anon.* (1973). Al-Anon Family Group Headquarters, Virginia Beach, VA.

2. Anonymous. (1985). *Today's Gift: Daily Meditations for Families.* Hazelden, Center City, MN.

3. Beattie, Melody. (1992). *Codependent No More: How to stop controlling others and start caring for yourself.* Hazelden, Center City, MN.

4. Beattie, Melody. (2009). *The New Codependency: Help and guidance for today's generation.* Simon & Schuster, New York, NY.

5. Beattie, Melody. (1990). *The Language of Letting Go: Hazelden meditation series.* Hazelden, Center City, MN.

6. Center for Nonviolent Communication. www.cnvc.org/Training/feelings-inventory.

7. Cermak, Timmen L. MD (1986). *Diagnosing and Treating Co-Dependence: A guide for professionals who work with chemical dependents, their spouses and children.* Johnson Institute Books, Minneapolis, MN.

8. Cloud, Henry & Townsend, John. (1992). *Boundaries: When to say yes, when to say no to take control of your life.* Zondervan, Grand Rapids, MI.

9. Cloud, Henry & Townsend, John (2003). *Boundaries Face to Face: How to have that difficult conversation you've been avoiding.* Zondervan, Grand Rapids, MI.

10. Cloud, Henry & Townsend, John (1995). *Safe People: How to find relationships that are good for you and avoid those that aren't.* Zondervan, Grand Rapids, MI.

11. Codependency Assessment. www.counselingctr.org/assessments/Codependency.doc.

12. Hay, Louise. (1984). *You Can Heal Your Life.* Hay House, Inc. Santa Monica, CA.

13. Hemfelt, Robert, Minirth, Frank, Meier, Paul. (1989). *Love is a choice: Recovery for codependent relationships.* Thomas Nelson Publishers, Nashville, TN.

14. Laaser, Mark, Ph.D. & Laaser, Debra. (2008). *The Seven Desires.* Zondervan, Grand Rapids, MI. Faithfulandtrue.com.

15. Mellody, Pia. (2003). *Facing Codependence: What it is, where it comes from, how it sabotages our lives.* HarperCollins, San Francisco, CA.

16. Nacoa. net/pdfs/addicted.pdf, National Association for Children of Alcoholics.

17. Schaef, Anne Wilson. (1986). *Co-dependence: Misunderstood-Mistreated.* Harper & Row, San Francisco, CA.

18. Shapiro, Francine, Ph.D. (2012). *Getting Past Your Past: Take control of your life with self-help techniques from EMDR.* Rodale Books, New York, NY.

19. Springle, Pat. (1977). *ER: Breaking free from the hurt and manipulation of dysfunctional relationships.* Rapha Publishing/Word, Inc., Houston/Dallas, TX.

20. Subby, Robert. (1987). *Lost in the Shuffle: The co-dependent reality.* Health Communications, Inc., Deerfield Beach, FL.

21. *The Journey of Recovery: A New Testament.* (2006). International Bible Society, Colorado Springs, CO.

22. Williams, G. (1998). *Adult Children of Alcoholics: Parental Bonding, Adult Attachment, and Spirituality,* A dissertation presented to the faculty of the California integral studies.

23. Wilson, Sandra D. (1990). *Released from Shame: Recovery for adult children of dysfunctional families.* InterVarsity Press, Downers Grove, IL.

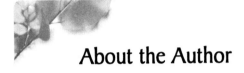

About the Author

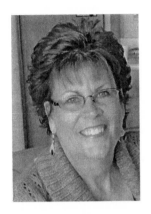

Peg Roberts, LMFT is a Licensed Marriage and Family Therapist, President and Clinical Director for her counseling practice, Spirit of Hope Counseling Center. She is also an approved Supervisor for the Minnesota Board of Marriage and Family Therapy and the AAMFT (American Association of Marriage and Family Therapy). She has been in the counseling field for over 15 years and has mentored and supervised many new therapists completing their LMFT, LPC and LPCC credentials. Also, she is certified in EMDR and working towards becoming an EMDR Consultant.

Spirit of Hope is a Christian Counseling Center and has several therapists collaborating with one another offering hope and healing to individuals, couples, families, and children. They are located in Minnetonka, MN and at Spiritofhopecc.com.

Peg lives in Excelsior, MN with her husband of 37 years. They have three grown children and five grandchildren and find their greatest joy in their family.

What Others Have to Say

"I loved the book! It was easy to read and extremely helpful – from the perspective of your everyday person. I read *Reclaiming a Lost Soul* not from a therapist's standpoint, but from the codependent's standpoint. The book was an amazing reminder of all the trials and dysfunction I lived in. I have worked very hard on my own codependency and addiction issues, and I realized there are more avenues waiting to come to light for everyone when they are ready. I had my own *Aha* moments and it helped me to remember some of the tools in my toolbox."

Anonymous

"Codependency is a topic that can affect anyone at anytime, without realizing what may be taking place or impacting our lives negatively. This book not only gives us examples of ways we can develop codependent behaviors, but also an understanding of what we can do to develop new and healthy ones. Peg did a wonderful job creating a book that anyone who picks it up to read can understand and relate to it. Thank you for putting your expertise and experiences into writing for us all to learn and grow."

Anonymous

.

CPSIA information can be obtained
at www.ICGtesting.com
Printed in the USA
FFOW05n1003010816